SUCCESS STORIES

"I loved every minute with you and your beautiful spirit. You gave me so much to think/work on, and I came home with this incredible calm all about me."

— **Jane Waterman**. Brisbane QLD

"I had a great session last Thursday with Kirstyn. She removed a number of blockages, and the main one that I had been working on was my feeling of nervousness. Four days later, and I'm still feeling great. Thanks, Kirstyn, for your help and words of wisdom."

— **Virginia Bergman**. Brisbane QLD

"Thank you for today's group session. I feel lighter and cleaner and can see now how far down I'd let myself get before reaching out for help. I have to remember what this feels like and maintain the higher vibration. It was a privilege to be blessed by your wonderful energy. I'm grateful that you're doing this important and valuable work."

— **Dianna King**. Melbourne VIC

Just spending time with Kirstyn is a calming experience; her attitude to life and the inevitable circumstances it brings is truly refreshing. She has learned some amazing, yet simple strategies for staying in control and calm in many situations. This isn't just head knowledge; this is wisdom that has come from experience and methods that work. The simple act of "remembering to breathe" and focusing on my heartbeat has been so helpful for me in many different situations. In our busy pressured lives, I thoroughly recommend making a habit of 'Remaining Calm in the Midst of Chaos'.

— **Melina Windolf**. Brisbane QLD

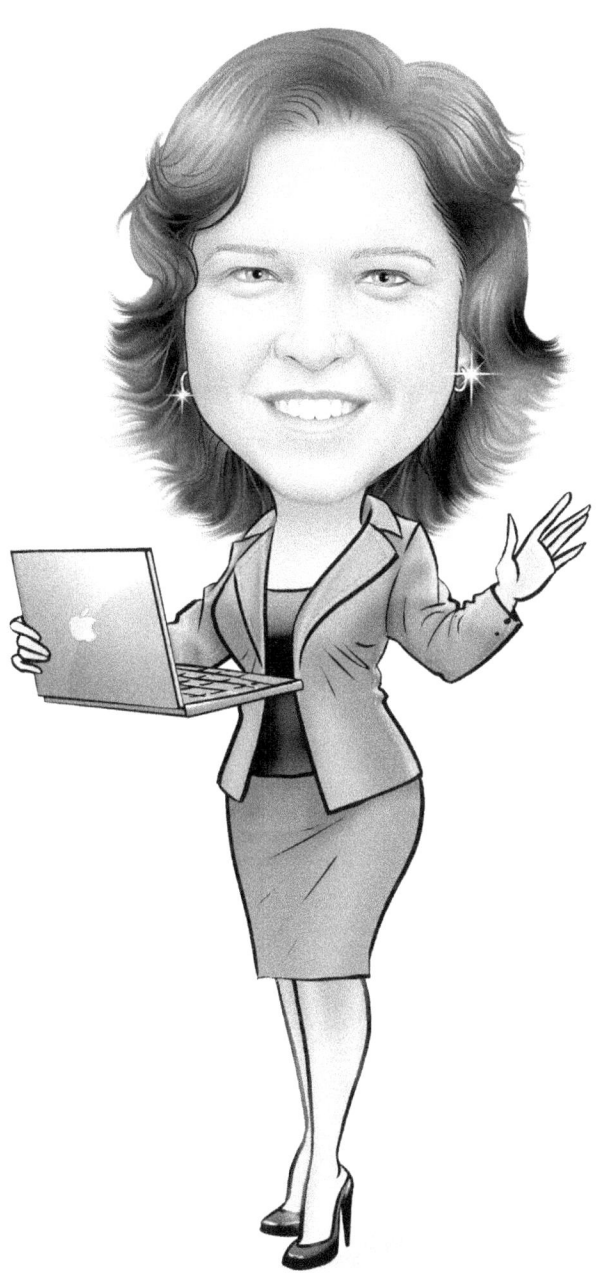

www.kirstynmarriott.com

How to Remain *Calm* in the Midst of *Chaos*

New Edition

KIRSTYN MARRIOTT

Copyright © 2017 Our Life Essentials

Published by Our Life Essentials
PO Box 3147 Brisbane, Queensland, Australia

All rights reserved.

Edited by Wendy Millgate, Wendy & Words

National Library of Australia Cataloguing-in-Publication entry
Creator: Marriott, Kirstyn, author.
Title: How to remain calm in the midst of chaos : a holistic guide
to a calmer balanced life / Kirstyn
Marriott ; Wendy Millgate, editor.
Edition: New Edition
Subjects: Stress (Psychology)--Prevention. Stress management. Calmness. Mind and body.
Other Creators/Contributors: Millgate, Wendy, editor.

ISBN: 978-0-9954189-0-5 (paperback)

Important Note to the Reader
The ideas, suggestions and techniques in this book should not be used to diagnose or treat any medical conditions nor be used in place of sound medical therapies and recommendations. Information contained in this book has been gathered from years of personal research and experience, and it is now practised in individual and group facilitation with great results. It is designed to provide helpful information on the subjects discussed. For diagnosis or treatment of any medical problem, consult your own physician.

The publisher and author are not responsible for any specific health or allergy needs that may require medical supervision and are not liable for any damages or negative consequences from any treatment, action, application or preparation, to any person reading or following the information in this book. References are provided for informational purposes only and do not constitute endorsement of any websites or other sources. Readers should be aware that the websites listed in this book may change.

Dedication

This book is dedicated to YOU, the reader. My aim is to help you live a happier, more productive life with emotional clarity.

Just as others have shared their knowledge with me, I now share my knowledge with you.

My hope and prayer is that this will be the end of your search or the beginning of a solution, as it was for me.

I hope you will act upon it and enjoy its fruits.

May God guide and guard your heart.

Contents

Preface	xi
Definitions	xvii
1. What is Stress?	1
2. How Our Words and Thoughts Affect Us	9
3. Stress and the Body	21
4. Food For Thought	29
5. Is Your System Overdue for a Tune Up?	39
6. Shifting Sizes	45
7. Harnessing the Subconcious Mind	55
8. Emotions! Are They Overrated?	63
9. Forgiveness! Seriously?	73
10. Essential Support	81
11. What is Lurking in our DNA?	87
12. Tapping Into New Life	93
Conclusion	97
Time for Reflection	100
Appendix	101
Acknowledgements	102
About the Author	104
References	106

Preface

The first time something bad happens to you, you're a victim. Each time after, you're a volunteer.

You may be a victim of your past, as all of us at some point are, and that's fine. We accepted beliefs passed down to us, and now we're not sure if that's really how we want to live.

Once the lights come on, and you understand acting on these beliefs isn't working for you, you're a volunteer in continuing, or discontinuing, what you know isn't working. That's when the first signs of awakening occur; you are now in the neighbourhood of the potential to change the whole course of your life.

When I look back over the past twenty-five years, I realise there were many times when I felt aspects of my life weren't working, and I made changes accordingly. Still it didn't seem enough. I suffered with unrelenting hormonal imbalance, constant stress and superwoman expectations (self-inflicted).

I also enrolled in a countless number of diets with great success, followed by great disappointment at not being able to maintain the loss. (I'm sure some of you can relate to that.) The older I got, the message coming through was, *This is what life is like.*

But I wasn't going to buy that for a minute. Who benefits if we're on a constant diet? Yes, diet companies. I knew there had to be a better way.

I believe that the body is a remarkable instrument, and given the right tools, it can do what it does best: keep you alive, happy and healthy. I've never been one who frequents fast food restaurants or eat out a lot. When you have a family of five, eating out regularly sure does drain the reserves. Food wasn't the issue behind my weight and health issues. I just had to find what was!

My hormones were so out of whack that each month I had a terrible time. It would take me weeks to recover, and then it would start all over again. I got rather impatient and began looking for answers.

I've always been a problem-solver and believe there's a better way, so I went to the doctors and did all of the tests to rule out anything sinister. It turns out my iron levels were extremely low, which didn't surprise me with what I'd been experiencing. I thought there needed to be a reason why I'd feel debilitated every month.

I went off to the gynaecologist to see if he could answer some questions. His solution was a hysterectomy! *Okay,* I thought. *Let's get it over and done with.*

Consciously, I was happy about it, as I thought my problems would be over. Yet my inner voice kept telling me that this wasn't the answer. Deep down I knew I wasn't addressing the cause, so I ditched the operation, put my detective hat on and said, 'Okay, God, what's the answer? Please point me in the right direction'.

As a HeartMath provider, I was blessed to have access to an abundance of research and resources. One day, as I was listening to a webinar by some of the team from HeartMath and Dr Sara Gottfried (gynaecologist), I learned that what I was experiencing physically was a manifestation of what I was experiencing emotionally: total *overwhelm*.

I was constantly worried about work, and family, and finances, which is pretty much a universal female issue. I was feeling fatigued, anxious, unsexy, fat and cranky (the last one not really, but my family said I was). I just didn't feel like my old self.

Dr Gottfried said, 'You should know there's a different way to live. You can feel delicious, vital and genuinely content. You can live an

PREFACE

extraordinary life, and you can feel great, regardless of your age, even if it sounds unlikely or unimaginable'.

I thought, *WOW!* She had me hanging on the edge of my seat.

She went on to say, 'It's easier to rebalance your hormones than to live with the misery of hormonal imbalance'.

It excited me to learn that it was possible to feel better in middle age than I did in my twenties as a perfect hormonal specimen, and that I didn't need to settle for imbalance, as it's not a natural state of being.

At this point, I was almost jumping up and down. All I could think was, *Thank you, God.* I had found the next piece of the puzzle.

Prior to becoming a HeartMath provider, and SimplyHealed and EFT practitioner, I studied Hypnotherapy and Neuro Linguistic Programming (NLP), as I was fascinated about why we do what we do and also why it's difficult to break bad habits.

By delving more into the subconscious mind, I became open to the reality that going over past situations makes you feel the emotions again as if it's happening for the first time. The body doesn't recognise if it's real or imagined, so it acts as if it is real, and a whole gamut of physiological processes kick in.

Now, that was an alarming thought, as I was becoming aware of what programs I was running that didn't serve my purpose and had overstayed their welcome. It was time to let it all go.

I read a story of a group of scientists who were studying a monkey species in the jungles of Africa. It was important to the scientists that the monkeys weren't harmed in the capture process. They devised a trap consisting of a small jar with a long, narrow neck, in which they placed a handful of nuts. The scientists then set out a certain number of these jars in various locations and returned to their campsite.

On discovering the nuts in the bottle, a monkey would thrust their hand into the long neck and grab a fistful. Then when they tried to pull their hand out, while still holding onto the nuts, they discovered their fist wouldn't pass through the narrow neck of the bottle. But even though they were unable to escape with their prize, they were unwilling to let it go.

You might be thinking how foolish those monkeys were! Yet, in some respects, we're just like them, clinging to the very things that hold us back, remaining captive through sheer unwillingness to let go.

For example, if we feel that a friend, work colleague or even a family member has treated us unjustly, we'll say, 'I can never forgive that person'. However, this says more about us than the person we feel we can't forgive.

If we step back and take an honest look at our life, we may find that we also hold on to things, much like the monkeys that continued to cling to those nuts, and they're keeping us trapped. It may be extra weight, negative judgement of others or ourselves, anger, fear, a toxic relationship or perhaps a job that's not right for us.

Many people spend their days complaining about being tied to a bottle, so to speak, and yet they're unwilling to let the belief, idea or person go, even when doing so would bring them the freedom they desire.

It might be time for you to take a few minutes to recognise what, if any, unhealthy patterns you're holding onto in your life. It's so liberating to finally recognise and release what's holding you back.

I have since gone on to learn more about emotional heritage and inherited issues. Just as we inherit our eye and hair colour, we can inherit emotional/energy baggage. Learning how to shed my own emotional baggage, and those trapped emotions, is transforming me back to the whole being God intended me to be.

When I found Certified Pure Therapeutic Grade (CPTG) essential oils back in 2014, I was amazed by the support these beautiful aromatic compounds gave me. I saw remarkable emotional transformations with my clients and family. I'd used other brands of essential oil in the past, but never had I seen such remarkable changes right before my eyes. Who

PREFACE

would have thought that one drop of oil could have such a profound effect on my emotions, physical body and mental health?

When my father passed away in February 2016, these essential oil blends brought much comfort in a distressing, heartbreaking and sad time. The blends I used as soon as I learnt of his death were *Comforting Blend*, *Renewing Blend* and *Reassuring Blend*. I continued to use this combo right up to his Celebration of Life service and felt their power and support. I was able to process my grief calmly and peacefully.

In bringing the information together in this book, I was reminded time and time again how complex we are and how finely tuned our body is. If we're out of balance in some area, it throws us off as a whole. We're constantly learning and growing, and we will never be perfect! However, we do have the choice to change how we live life. Money isn't what makes us wealthy; it's our minds and life choices.

When we're grateful and appreciate the good things we have now, and know that's where our happiness lies rather than thinking of what we don't have, that's true contentment. Only then will our problems seem conquerable and our stress levels manageable.

Now is the time to go out there and be the person you really are! You can do it.

God bless you!

DEFINITIONS

Chaos
Noun
Complete disorder and confusion.
Behaviour so unpredictable as to appear random, owing to great sensitivity to small changes in conditions
Synonyms: confusion, disorder, mess, clutter, muddle, welter.

Calm
Adjective
(Of a person, action, or manner) Not showing or feeling nervousness, anger, or other emotions
Noun
The absence of violent or confrontational activity within a place or group.
Verb
Make (someone) tranquil and quiet; soothe
Synonyms
Adjective
quiet, tranquil, still, placid, serene, peaceful
Noun
quiet, calmness, quietness, tranquillity, serenity
Verb
pacify, quiet, appease, soothe, lull, quieten

"What I am suggesting is that each of us turn from the negativism that permeates our society and look for the remarkable good among those with whom we associate, that we speak of one another's virtues more than we speak of one another's faults, that optimism replace pessimism, that our faith exceed our fears. When I was a young man and was prone to speak critically, my father would say: 'Cynics do not contribute, sceptics do not create, doubters do not achieve.'"

— Gordon B. Hinckley

1

What is Stress?

Stress has become the number one malady of our time. The constant pressure associated with living in a fast-paced world has created an environment where nearly everyone feels its effects.

Stress is a term used to describe the wear and tear the body experiences in reaction to major happenings like illness, injury, career and lifestyle changes. But even the minor hassles can cause pressure and tension. Peak-hour traffic, waiting in line and too many emails can often do the most damage.

Stress is the body and mind's response to any pressure that disrupts the normal balance. It occurs when our perception of events doesn't meet expectations, and we're unable to manage our reaction. Stress will express itself as resistance, tension, strain or frustration that throws off our physiological and psychological equilibrium, thus keeping us out of sync. If our equilibrium is disturbed for too long, the stress can become disabling and create numerous health problems.

Stress and its effects are often misunderstood. We look at outside events as the source, but the real cause is our emotional reactions to them. The stress we experience in today's world often goes unnoticed and unmanaged. Many people have simply adapted to it in an unhealthy way, resigned to thinking 'this is just the way it is'. Unfortunately, lack of stress management has created a pandemic of low-grade anxiety and depression.

For years, I pushed through each change; I guess you could say I adapted. If there were times where I felt I needed a change, I would have a massage or go on holidays. However, over time I would still react the same way whenever a stressful situation would present itself, as I hadn't learned any skills to assist me in handling the situation.

I started to question why I was always feeling tired and had no real motivation. Though I always got things done, I think it was more out of a sense of duty to adhere to the conventional way of living.

On starting to do some research, I became alarmed that there were so many others like myself, struggling with low energy, lack of motivation, being constantly run down and on the rollercoaster of accepting, *This is just the way it is*.

It made me wonder, *What's going on?*

The answer is that the central nervous system controls stress. The hypothalamus serves as a central processing unit for the whole brain. It has connections to all of the limbic systems, which are the emotional centres of the brain. In fact, it has nerve connections to virtually every part of the brain and connects to the rest of our body through the hormones that it manufactures and releases through the pituitary.

This list of ten functions will give you an idea of some of the power the hypothalamus has. In no particular order, they are:

1 : WHAT IS STRESS?

- arterial blood pressure
- sex organ function
- thyroid hormone function
- body temperature
- regulation of body water by thirst and kidney function
- uterine contraction
- breast milk production
- adrenal gland function
- emotional drive
- growth hormone levels

Physiologically, stress can result in huge changes to these responses, especially in glucose, insulin, adrenaline, cortisol (the stress hormone) and growth hormone levels. Stress does have its place. It gets us out of bed in the morning and gives the body a burst of cortisol. However, if we've depleted our reserves from the previous days and weeks, this task becomes increasingly difficult.

After digesting that information, it occurred to me that to effectively relieve stress, I had to understand it's not external events or situations that do the harm; it's how we respond to those events. More precisely, it's our feelings about the event that determines whether there are negative effects of stress or if we can ultimately relieve it.

Emotions or feelings have a powerful impact on the human body. Frustration, insecurity and depressing feelings are stressful and inhibit optimal health and relief from stress. Positive emotions like appreciation, care and love not only feel good, they promote health, performance and well-being.

Now, most of us are inclined to focus on the negative and dwell on what we're not happy about. Creating a base of worry and anxiety leads to an immune system that won't function at peak performance.

Stress often starts with a feeling. You first experience tension or worry, and then it escalates into stronger emotions of frustration, anxiety or anger. Finally, you end up overloaded and exhausted.

"We are our choices." — Jean-Paul Sartre

In our society, we don't always like to acknowledge feelings, because if we do, and admit to ourselves that emotions are managing us rather than the other way around, we may fear we're incapable, or even crazy. We tend to bottle them up and not admit we're hurting or feeling bad.

The truth is that our emotions are running us ragged, and deep inside we can feel the volcano slowly bubbling up, but instead of dealing with it, we ignore it, squish it, hide it and take it out on others or even blame them for the way we feel.

If we can't find relief, we either blow up or become reclusive, taking ourselves out of circulation. This is what's commonly termed the 'fight-or-flight' response.

The stress then triggers the brain circuits and hormones to prepare the body to protect itself for a dangerous situation. The real problem is that we need these processes to take place, so we can survive in a dangerous situation.

However, with everyday situations triggering these responses, we get to the stage where we're overloaded. We go off at the slightest inconvenience such as a traffic jam or a looming deadline. I'm sure you can recall many times where you maybe overreacted. The great news is…

IT DOESN'T HAVE TO BE THIS WAY!

1 : WHAT IS STRESS?

"The real voyage of discovery consists not in seeking new landscapes, but having new eyes." — Marcel Proust

Stress can also be felt when too few demands are made, such as when people feel bored, undervalued or under-stimulated, whether at work and at home, with the latter being the more frequent cause.

The effects of pressure at any time can be offset by a number of differing factors: more sleep, support systems in the home or work environment, an individual's personality or the use of coping strategies. Stress could be viewed as the balance between the pressures and these varied factors.

People have different reactions to stress. What may be too much pressure for one person at a specific time may not be for another, or even that same person, at a different time.

The signs of stress

It's important to spot the signs of stress in others and ourselves. Some of the symptoms are:

Emotional

- lack of confidence
- lack of self-esteem
- feeling out of control
- lack of motivation
- anger
- frustration
- feeling defensive
- being overly sensitive to criticism
- becoming easily tearful

- irritability
- mood swings

Physical
- frequent colds/infections
- allergies/rashes/skin irritations
- constipation/diarrhoea/IBS
- weight loss or gain
- indigestion/heartburn/ulcers
- hyperventilating/lump in the throat/pins and needles
- dizziness/palpitations
- panic attacks/nausea
- physical tiredness
- menstrual changes/loss of libido/sexual problems
- heart problems/high blood pressure
- aches/pains and muscle tension/grinding teeth

Mental
- inability to concentrate or make simple decisions
- memory lapses
- vagueness
- easily distracted
- less intuitive and creative
- worrying
- negative thinking
- depression and anxiety

Behavioural
- no time for relaxation or pleasurable activities
- prone to accidents or forgetfulness

1 : WHAT IS STRESS?

- increased reliance on alcohol, smoking, caffeine, recreational or illegal drugs
- becoming a workaholic
- poor time management and/or inferior standards of work
- absenteeism
- self-neglect / change in appearance
- social withdrawal
- relationship problems
- insomnia or waking tired
- recklessness
- aggressive/angry outbursts
- uncharacteristically lying

When I looked through the list, a number of them popped up I thought were just normal life events that would pass with time. However, looking back, I can see more issues on the list showing up in my life, thus compounding my stress symptoms. It was time to take action!

On our journey of self-discovery, it's crucial to recognise when something isn't working and acknowledge that we have the power to change it. Sometimes it seems easier just to live with our bad habits rather than having to bring forth the courage to do something about it. Often the process of letting go is what leads us to something better.

"You are essentially who you create yourself to be, and all that occurs in your life is the result of your own making."
— Stephen Richards

Time for Reflection

In what areas of your life have you noticed four or more stress symptoms showing up?

Are these symptoms triggered by particular events or circumstances?

2

How Our Words and Thoughts Affect Us

The phrase I hear all the time is, 'You're going to eat those words'. But what does that really mean? My understanding is that what we say not only affects others but also affects ourselves. Words are wonderful when used in a proper way. They can encourage, edify and give confidence to the hearer. The right word spoken at the right time can actually be life changing. However, the same can be said regarding an inappropriate or negative word.

We can literally increase our own joy by using kind and happy words. We can also upset ourselves by talking unnecessarily about our problems or events and people who've hurt us. I'm sure, like me, you've had situations where something negative happened to you, and your friends, with all good intentions, continued asking about it.

What happens each time you tell the story is that it keeps bringing that emotion back to the surface, when all you want to do is move on and get over it. What happened is a part of your life, and there's no denying that. However, if you know how to take the emotion out of the ordeal, you will have more clarity with that situation, and it won't keep haunting you forever and a day.

When we understand the power of words and realise that we can choose what we think and speak, our lives can be transformed. Our words aren't forced on us; they formulate in our thoughts, and then we speak them. We can learn to choose our thoughts, to resist wrong, or toxic, ones and think only on those that are good, healthy and life-driven.

Anyone who wants to be healthy is careful to choose quality food that will provide good nutrition. If we want to be healthy in our body, soul and spirit, we should also choose to take in words and thoughts that build us up and increase our peace and joy. We can rightfully say our words and thoughts are food for our body and soul.

> *"The greatest weapon against stress is our ability to choose one thought over another."* — William James

Let's take a look at how our physiology is affected by our thoughts and words.

Changing our brain and body

Every time you have a thought, it's actively changing your brain and your body...for better or worse. A thought may seem harmless, but should it become toxic, it can be physically, emotionally or spiritually dangerous.

2 : HOW OUR WORDS AND THOUGHTS AFFECT US

Advances in psychoneuroimmunology and neuroscience have shed more light on this area in recent years.

Psychoneuroimmunology is the science that looks at the three-way collaboration in the body where psychology sets off neurological changes that in turn can affect immunity. This science shows us how we not only affect our health through our thoughts, we can alter its direction by interceding and altering our thoughts as we process our emotional responses.

When stressed, depressed, angry, anxious or feeling guilty, we're more prone to misinterpreting events and thinking in a distorted way. One distorted thought tends to lead to another, and before long we're trapped in a downward spiral, This is where neuroscience supports the concept of our ability to change our thoughts and alter our brain.

I find neuroscience fascinating!

So what is it?

Neuroscience, the study of the nervous system, advances the understanding of human thought, emotion and behaviour. Neuroscientists use tools ranging from computers to special dyes to examine molecules, nerve cells, networks, brain systems and behaviour. From these studies, they learn how the nervous system develops and functions normally and what goes wrong in neurological disorders.

Cognitive neuroscientists study functions such as perception and memory in animals by using behavioural methods and other neuroscience techniques. In humans, they use non-invasive brain scans, such as Positron Emission Tomography and Magnetic Resonance Imaging, to uncover routes of neural processing that occur during language use, problem solving and other tasks.

Behavioural neuroscientists study the processes underlying behaviour in humans and animals. Their tools include microelectrodes, which measure electrical activity of neurons, and brain scans that show the parts of the brain that are active during activities such as seeing, speaking or remembering.

The neuroscience of today has debunked many myths about what was previously believed about the brain. As an example, it's not true that we use only ten percent, or less, of our brains.

The ability of the brain to recreate itself as a flexible network of neuronal connection has become more well documented and is now recognised under the term 'neuroplasticity'. Our minds seem to be powerful enough to shape and reshape our brains, depending on what we focus on. It has, for example, been documented by researchers at University College London that their black cab drivers who 'learn' the streets of London and don't rely on a navigation system, have a significantly larger hippocampus as compared to the rest of the population.

The hippocampus is the part of the brain that manages spacial orientation. Since it's under constant demand by its users, in this example meaning the cab drivers, it has grown much like a muscle bulks up when trained and used regularly.

In other words, it's fair to assume the opposite is true as well, and if we continue to let our mind respond to stimulation with stressful reactive patterns, it will reinforce the circuits and biochemical cascades that lead to chronic stress.

We can empower ourselves to shift into strong ownership of our brain and learn to change its state to be powerful in front of the stress response.

So let's see what's been discovered regarding our thoughts and words.

What actually goes on?

Thoughts are measurable and occupy mental 'real estate'. They're active, which means they grow and change. Thoughts influence every decision, word, action and physical reaction we make.

The result of toxic thinking translates into stress in your body, and this type of stress is far more than just a fleeting emotion. Stress is a global term for the extreme strain on your body's system as a result of toxic thinking. It harms the body and the mind in a magnitude of ways, from

2 : HOW OUR WORDS AND THOUGHTS AFFECT US

patchy memory to poor mental health, and problems with the immune system, heart and digestion (as listed in the previous chapter).

Feelings turning into chemical responses in our brain stops cells from reacting to what you express and believe. They document information and can even build new neural pathways (highways of information). Body chemistry can become acidic, and you need an alkaline body to stay healthy.

The human brain is comprised of a variety of parts that all function as a whole to process the information it receives. The primary section accountable for processing is referred to as the reptilian brain. The second brain is the limbic system, often known as the emotional brain. We can reach the limbic system with the use of images.

An important part of the limbic system, the amygdala, evaluates the emotional benefit of stimuli. It's the primary part of the brain connected to anxious reactions, including the 'fight-flight-freeze' approach. The amygdala doesn't react to visuals or sound—just to scent. So as a way to manage the stress response, it's a good idea to use Certified Pure Therapeutic Grade essential oils, which affect the olfactory system and could be the difference between a quicker recovery and transition and a compromised immune state.

No system of the body is spared when stress is running rampant. Numerous research studies collectively show that up to eighty percent of physical, emotional and mental health issues today could be a direct result of our thoughts. WOW! Now if that doesn't wake you up, I'm not sure what will.

But there is hope! You can break the cycle of toxic thinking and start building healthy patterns that will bring peace to a stormy life.

Notice your thoughts.

I invite you right now to have a thought, any thought, related to a feeling, such as anger, sadness, inspiration, joy … Notice any changes in your body. You changed you. All thoughts, whether they be *I'm not good enough* or *I love you*, have the same measurable effects.

As you sit there, keep in mind that your body is undergoing numerous dynamic changes, triggered by your most recent thought. Did you know that your pancreas and adrenal glands were already busy secreting a few new hormones? Like a sudden lightning storm, different areas of your brain just surged with increased electrical current, releasing a stack of neurochemicals that are too numerous to name.

Your spleen and thymus gland sent out a mass email to your immune system to make a few modifications. Several different gastric juices started flowing. Your liver began processing enzymes that weren't present moments before you had the thought. Your heart rate fluctuated, your lungs altered their stroke volume, and blood flow to the capillaries in your hands and feet changed. All from just thinking one thought.

You are so very powerful!

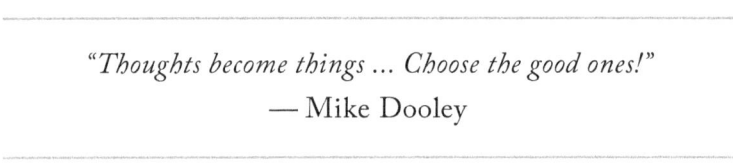

"Thoughts become things … Choose the good ones!"
— Mike Dooley

So how are you capable of performing all of those actions? You probably know already that the brain can manage and regulate many diverse functions throughout the body, but how responsible are we for the job our brain is doing as CEO of our body? Whether we like it or not, once a thought happens in the brain, the rest is history. All of the bodily reactions that occur from both our intentional or unintentional thinking unfold behind the scenes of our awareness. It's startling to realise how influential and extensive the effects of one or two conscious or unconscious thoughts can be.

Those seemingly unconscious thoughts that run through our mind daily, and repeatedly, create a cascade of chemical reactions that produce not only *what* we feel but also *how* we feel. The long-term effect of

2 : HOW OUR WORDS AND THOUGHTS AFFECT US

habitual thinking causes the body to move into a state of imbalance, or what's known as '*dis*-ease'.

Moment by moment, we train our body to be unhealthy through our repeated thoughts and reactions. By thinking, we cause our internal chemistry to be bumped out of the normal range so often, that the body's self-regulation system eventually redefines these abnormal states as normal and regular. It's a subtle process that maybe you've never given much attention to until now.

The surprising truth is that every single thought, whether positive or negative, goes through the same cycle when it forms. Thoughts are basically electrical impulses, chemicals and neurons. They look like a tree with branches. As the thoughts expand and become permanent, more branches grow, and the connections become stronger.

When you're under extreme stress and have intense feelings, chemicals flood your body and create physical effects. When those feelings are, for example, anger, fear, anxiety or bitterness, the effects on your health are nothing short of horrific in the long term.

Stress chemicals can be the kind of guests that don't know when they've overstayed their welcome. If they remain because your system is imbalanced, eventually they will tunnel deep inside the recesses of your mind, literally becoming part of who you are.

We've been experiencing the effects of all of our thoughts our entire lives and may not even know it. In the wake of a difficult time or stress in my life, I would break out in cold sores or have an upset tummy. I didn't make the connection at first and figured it was a coincidence. But now I know that more than likely it was the thoughts I'd adopted that were taking a toll on my health.

People who wish the flu on themselves always amaze me. They program it by saying, 'Every winter I get the flu'. One friend says they get it a couple of times, and they're never disappointed.

The lesson here is that your thoughts are powerful.

Thoughts create changes right down to the genetic levels, restructuring the cells' makeup. Scientists have shown that this restructuring is how disease is able to take hold of the body.

Thoughts aren't only scientifically measurable; we can verify them in our own bodies as well. We can feel them through our emotions. Healthy, non-toxic thoughts nurture and create a positive foundation in the neural networks of the mind. They strengthen positive chain reactions and release bio-chemicals, such as endorphins and serotonin, from the brain's natural pharmacy. Bathed in these positive environments, intellect flourishes, and with it, mental and physical health.

"To change the world takes time; to change yourself takes courage." — R.S. Low

Essential Oils Toolbox:

The most amazing combination of oils that support you to transform your thoughts in the stress response are CPTG *Calming Blend, Ylang Ylang, Comforting Blend, Wild Orange Oil* and *Lavender Oil.*

Exercise: Letting go of negative baggage

A great exercise to let go of negative baggage is to take yourself to a quiet, comfortable location, close your eyes and take three deep, cleansing breaths.

Keep the breathing going while you mentally scan all of the different areas of your life. Observe if/where any uncomfortable feelings arise.

2 : HOW OUR WORDS AND THOUGHTS AFFECT US

Pause yourself (in your mind) and ask, *Is this a situation I can let go of and have peace of mind about?*

Picture your life without this negativity in it. Hold that picture in your mind's eye.

Visualise those grey, cloudy, negative emotions loosening on every inhalation, and leaving your body and your energy on every exhalation.

During this process, remind yourself that it's always safe to let go of negative thoughts and emotions by saying, 'It is safe for me to let go'.

Tell yourself, *I am worthy and deserving of having a life without these shadows. I am worthy and deserving of this positive picture I am holding in my mind.*

Visualise clean, white light coming in to replace where those grey clouds had been.

Be open to receiving a life without the negative baggage.

It's okay if some emotion comes up during this process, but letting go doesn't have to be painful. Your spirit knows all of the details of the situation, and you've most likely already experienced many painful emotions along with it, so you don't need to revisit them all again.

Simply let go. Don't make it harder than that.

Release your grip. Surrender!

If you're anything like me, you probably have a number of areas where you will need to do this. If so, repeat the process as often as needed.

By letting go, you'll not only change how you see the situation, you have literally raised the energy of it.

Once you've removed the tethers, you will open up and move forward with the positive intentions of what you really want in life.

So where do we go after we recognise the problem and let go of the negative thoughts and emotions?

Our subconscious mind doesn't like a void. If we don't fill it after the release of negative thoughts and emotions, we take the chance of subconsciously filling it with more of the same. Therefore, it just makes sense to consciously replace lower energy with higher energy. That means we choose to no longer think the negative thoughts and instead focus on good, positive affirmations.

Writing your own positive affirmations is quite simple. By thinking of what it is you want to change in your life and how it would look in your 'ideal' world, you already have the basis of a great affirmation. Ask yourself, *How do I wish it was? How would I like it to be?* Your answers can easily be tweaked into the perfect affirmations for you.

Notice your speech patterns, and change them when necessary. For instance, do you ever say things like…

'I'm not good enough.'

'I can't afford it.'

'I'm so fat.'

'There are no good men/women out there for me.'

'I never have enough time to get things done.'

'The kids are always driving me crazy.'

All of these are examples of limited thinking. When you hear the negative self-talk creeping into your thoughts, acknowledge it briefly and then let it go by replacing it with a new, positive affirmation.

'I am always good enough.'

'Money flows to me. I always have more than enough.'

'I am worthy and deserving of a great life.'

'I love my healthy, fit body.'

'I am worthy of a healthy, happy relationship.'

'My kids are calm and balanced.'

Always state them in the present tense. I like to begin with 'I AM.' Even if you're thirty kilograms overweight, say, "I am at my healthy goal weight." Though your conscious mind isn't quite buying the positive affirmation, the subconscious mind, which sees in pictures, will believe it

2 : HOW OUR WORDS AND THOUGHTS AFFECT US

without question, and your behaviours will align with that subconscious belief. (I go deeper into the subconscious mind in *chapter 7*.)

If you catch yourself reverting back to any negative thought habits, ask yourself, *If I could have anything I want in this situation, what would that look like?* Feel it, smell it, taste it, touch it. The more senses you engage, the easier it becomes to manifest it into reality. The more vigilant you are about immediately kicking out those negative thoughts and replacing them with positive affirmations, the easier it becomes to make this your new mode of operation. It will become easier and easier to send away self-doubt as soon as it shows up, instead of allowing it to stay long enough to discourage you. With patience and practice, it becomes a habit, and that's how you re-weave your thought patterns into a beautiful tapestry.

If it's still difficult to budge some emotional baggage, look for a practitioner in emotional clearing to lead you through the process.

"Always think extra hard before crossing over to a bad side. If you were weak enough to cross over, you may not be strong enough to cross back!" — Victoria Addino

Time for Reflection

What are some of your most dominant thoughts in different areas of your life?

Are they predominantly critical?

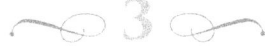

Stress and the Body

When we understand the mechanics of stress, we have the advantage of becoming more aware of, and sensitive to, our own stress levels and knowing when and how to take proactive steps. This increased awareness also helps our relationships with our family, friends and colleagues.

5 facts About Stress

Here are five facts about stress most people may not be aware of.

1. **Your body doesn't care if it's a big stress or little one**
   Our body doesn't discriminate between a BIG stress or a small one. No matter what the significance, stress affects the body in a predictable way, whether it's something major like the death of a close friend,

family member or even a pet, or something minor, like being cut off in traffic. There are 1400 biochemical events cascading through us with a typical stress reaction, which most people experience multiple times each day. Ignoring these reactions will bring on premature aging, cognitive function (brain function, thinking) will become impaired, and our energy will drain along with our effectiveness and clarity.

2. **Stress can make smart people do stupid things**
   According to brain researchers, stress causes cortical inhibition. This phenomenon helps to explain why smart people do dumb things. Put simply, stress inhibits a small part of the brain, which reduces the capacity to function at our best. To have the brain, heart and nervous system working in harmony we need to operate in a state of coherence, which means we're cognitively sharp, emotionally calm, and feel and think with enhanced clarity. Coherence facilitates cognitive functioning, where we're operating at peak performance mentally, emotionally and physically.

3. **People can become numb to their stress**
   We can become so accustomed to stress that we can be experiencing the physiological symptoms of it and yet be mentally numb from it. When we become well adapted to the daily pressures, irritations and annoyances that life can bring, it starts to appear normal.

   As small stresses accumulate quickly and sneak up on us, we may not realise how much they're reducing our mental and emotional clarity and influencing our overall health, until it shows up as a bad decision, an overreaction to a simple situation or an unwanted or unexpected diagnosis.

4. **We can control how we respond to stress**
   There are simple, scientifically validated solutions to stress that empower people to rewire their own stress response. Therefore, we can

let go of being victims of our own emotions, thoughts and attitudes. When we control how we respond to stress, we become more sensitive to stressful situations and the ways they're affecting us. We have the ability to implement the strategies to change it before they manifest as a physical, mental or emotional complaint.

5. **The best strategy is to handle stress in the moment**
Every time you find yourself in a stressful situation, deal with it right there in the moment. The 'binge and purge' approach when it comes to stress is not a successful way to deal with the situation; however, millions of people use this method. So we stress all day, believing we can wait until later to recover when we stop by a yoga class or the gym or take the weekend off.

Unfortunately, when we put off activating our own inner balance, our bodies have already activated the stress response, as well as all of the chemical reactions that go with it, and our health suffers.

HeartMath's research shows how emotions change our heart rhythm. Positive emotions create coherent heart rhythms, which look like rolling hills. It's a smooth and ordered pattern.

In contrast, negative emotions create chaotic, erratic patterns. Using a heart rhythm monitor, you can actually see your heart rhythms change in real time as you shift from stressful emotions, like anger and anxiety, to positive feelings like care or appreciation. *(See Diagram 1.)*

Coherent heart rhythm patterns facilitate higher brain function, whereas negative emotions inhibit a person's ability to think clearly. Coherent heart rhythms also create a feeling of solidarity and security.

HOW TO REMAIN CALM IN THE MIDST OF CHAOS

What Stress Does to Your Body

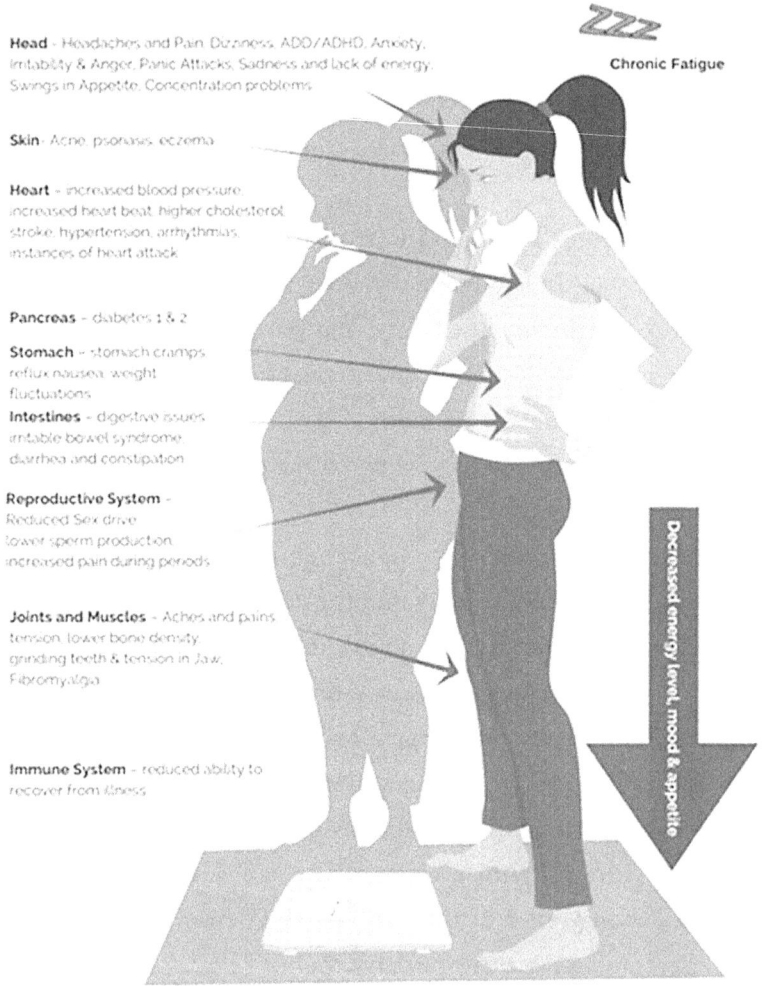

Diagram 1

"Stress is the trash of modern life – we all generate it, but if you don't dispose of it properly, it will pile up and overtake your life." — Terri Guillemets

---

3 : STRESS AND THE BODY

Human beings were designed to move, not sit on chairs. Therefore, exercise is an essential part of healthy the body's function. The good news is that exercise is your shortest route to a feeling of wellbeing and a physical glow.

Everyone knows that exercise is good for you and that it's one of the best stress combatants available. However, the number one excuse people give as to why they don't exercise is that they're too busy and stressed to fit it into their routine.

It can be easy to fall into that thought process, as well as a challenge to push yourself out of it, but you know if you stick with that belief cycle, you will always find justification for not taking action.

Not only does exercise keep the heart healthy and get oxygen into the system, it also helps deplete stress hormones and release mood-enhancing chemicals, such as endorphins, that help us better cope with stress.

Endorphins are often classified as the 'happy hormones'. Any form of physical activity leads to the release of these feel-good neurotransmitters. The increase in endorphins in your body leads to a feeling of euphoria, modulation of appetite, the release of different sex hormones and an enhancement of immune response. As result, you'll better be able to combat the negative effects of stress.

Whether you're building muscle or stamina, all types of exercise relax tense muscles and tissue. These can strongly contribute to stress-related aches and pains, such as neck or back problems and headaches.

Exercise is also particularly good when it's competitive, because it enables you to raise your game to a higher performance level than you would otherwise achieve. Try a sport with an opponent, such as tennis or badminton, or a situation where you can set up a race, such as cycling or swimming. You can even try power walking or jogging with a friend.

Exercise not only helps increase metabolism, but also spin off and clear mental fog and tension accumulated from anxiety, anger and worry.

The positive endorphins that exercise releases will also help you maintain a more positive outlook for a long time afterwards.

Avoid alcohol, nicotine and caffeine as coping mechanisms. Alcohol may seem to reduce the symptoms of stress, but abuse of it can cause anxiety as it wears off and eventually lead to dependence. It's also a depressant, so if you're feeling blue, it will only make the situation worse.

Similarly, drinking caffeine and smoking when you're feeling stressed and overwhelmed may seem calming, but these are powerful stimulants leading to higher—not lower—levels of stress and anxiety.

Stress and worry cause insomnia, and a lack of sleep can leave you vulnerable to even more stress.

It's much easier to keep your emotional balance if well rested, which is a key factor in coping with job and workplace stress. Try to improve the quality of your rest by keeping a sleep schedule and aiming for eight hours a night.

Essential Oils Toolbox:

Place a drop of Vetiver essential oil under your big toes to calm the mind before sleep.

I use this method, and twenty minutes later, I have trouble keeping my eyes open.

According to the Heartmath Institute:

'When we have plenty of energy, we can handle anything without experiencing stress. If we lack energy, even the slightest demands can cause us to become stressed. If you increase your energy, you increase your capacity for life and you are more positive and confident. You can handle more challenges and feel satisfied, because you are able to handle your life better. You experience more, achieve more and enjoy life more.'

3 : STRESS AND THE BODY

> *"The power behind taking responsibility for your actions lie in putting an end to negative thought patterns. You no longer dwell on what went wrong or focus on whom you are going to blame. You don't waste time building roadblocks to your success. Instead, you are set free and can now focus on succeeding."* — Lorii Myers

Once a person engages a positive emotion, there's an obvious change on the heart rate monitor. *(Diagram 2.)* I see it all the time when I have a client on the monitor. The realisation that they have the ability to change their physiology in a heartbeat, and they don't need to bathe in misery, is a light bulb moment.

Emotional State Heart Rhythm

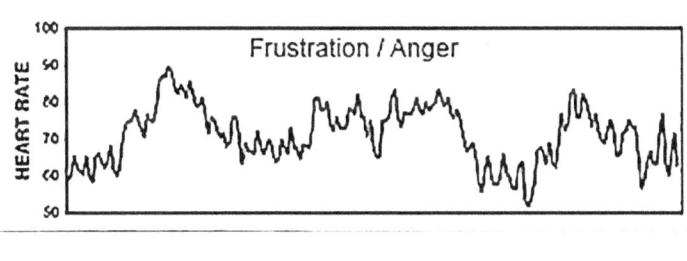

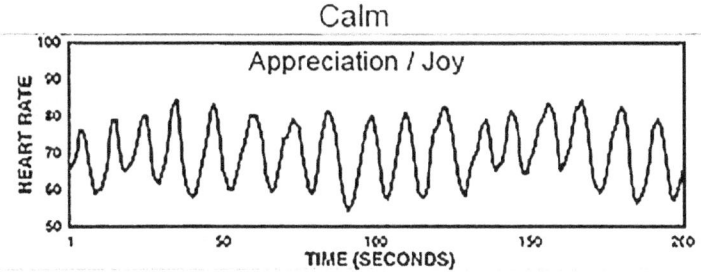

Diagram 2

Some of the non-physical issues that control the physiology of your body are memories, beliefs, actions and thoughts. They can kick the body's stress response into action when is shouldn't be.

It shuts off the cells and the immune system, so in the end we wind up with every kind of health problem imaginable. Both the physical and non-physical problems all originate from heart issues or cellular memories that create destructive energy frequencies, which send our body into a false stress response.

When you decide to deal with your heart issues, your cellular memories, and remove drama from your life, you will have the ability to fulfil your dreams of having a great career, peak performance, good health, and positive relationships with everyone in your life.

You enhance your life by understanding the importance of healing the source of your heart issues, and the destructive, often painful, cellular memories that contain false beliefs.

Time for Reflection

In which of your activities do you feel you're not at your cognitive best?

Do you binge and purge on so-called stress-buster activities and find you haven't achieved the desired result?

What, if any, health challenges are you experiencing?

If you do experience these challenges, do you feel there's a link between it and your chosen stress-busting actions?

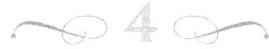

Food For Thought

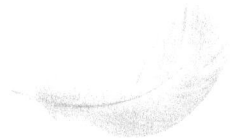

Make food choices that keep you sustained. Even the task of eating can bring on the stress response in the body. Worrying about what you should or shouldn't eat sends signals to the body that dictate how to respond to the food you're consuming.

If your mind/body believes it's at war, it will store fat as a protective response to stress and the fear of possible starvation. It's no wonder people have a difficult time losing weight and keeping it off.

If you're struggling with weight issues, is it possible this is what's going on with you? Low blood sugar can make you feel anxious and irritable, while eating too much has a lethargic effect. Healthy eating can help you get through stressful workdays. By eating small but frequent meals, you can help your body maintain an even level of blood sugar, keep your energy up, stay focused and avoid mood swings.

Caffeine

First thing in the morning, the alarm goes off, and we drag ourselves from a restful state before reaching for our first cup of caffeine and probably some highly processed food, such as toast or sugar-loaded cereals. However, by the time we reach work, that sugary cereal may have shut down our immune system. The body can only function efficiently with about three teaspoons of sugar in the bloodstream at any given time. Anything exceeding this amount, and our immune system may be suppressed for up to six hours.

Our body is also now on high alert, thanks to the caffeine, which stays in the body for six hours or more before it starts to diminish, the whole time triggering the release of cortisol, which prepares us for fight or flight and compounds our stress problem. More coffee consumed during this time increases the release of cortisol.

One of the first steps to managing stress and improving sleep quality is eliminating caffeine. Australians consume an average of 230 mg of caffeine a day—similar levels to those consumed in the USA and Canada.

The amount of caffeine in tea and coffee depends on how strong you make it. Below is a rough guide:

Tea (250ml) 10–50mg
Decaf instant coffee (250ml) 3mg
Instant coffee (250ml) 60–80mg
Percolated/plunger coffee (250ml) 60–120mg
Cola-type soft drinks (250ml) 36 mg
'Energy' drinks (375ml) 80 mg
Hot chocolate (1 cup) 6 mg
Milk chocolate (100g) 20 mg
Dark chocolate (30g) 20 mg

4 : FOOD FOR THOUGHT

Although most people can handle these amounts, there's a huge variation in the rate at which we detoxify stimulants like caffeine. Genetic variations in the liver enzyme that breaks it down means some people can eliminate caffeine quickly, while for others it may take as much as twelve to twenty-four hours for full elimination of the caffeine from a single cup of coffee.

Anyone who has trouble sleeping should simply try caffeine avoidance for seven to ten days. This has to be strict, so not just coffee but tea, chocolate, drugs with caffeine and energy drinks should be included.

A great way to kick start your liver after a night's sleep is to consume a large glass of warm water with half a cup of lime juice in it. I often add a drop of dōTERRA's lime or lemon essential oil to my morning warm water, which is a great way to get those cells hydrated and the body systems kicking in for the day.

Alcohol

Alcohol should also be eliminated in people with regular insomnia. It causes the release of adrenaline and disrupts the production of serotonin (an important brain chemical that initiates sleep). When you don't get enough sleep, it drives down Leptin levels, which means you don't feel as satisfied after you eat. Leptin is a hormone made by fat cells that decreases your appetite.

Lack of sleep also causes ghrelin levels to rise. Ghrelin, or GHR, is a growth hormone-releasing peptide that increases appetite and plays a role in body weight. This means your appetite is stimulated, so you want more food. Not a great combination.

'White' foods

'White' food is often heavily processed and refined, resulting in poor nutritional value for the calories you consume. This includes white breads, pastas, many cereal products, and even cracker-type snacks marketed as healthy and low fat. Think about some other white staples too, like flour, and even processed milk and cheese products. They spike insulin and stress hormone levels. Some white foods that are okay to eat are natural and non-processed, like cauliflowers, rice, potato, fish and chicken.

When stressed, we reach for quick fixes—stimulants like coffee or foods high in fat or sugar. Nevertheless, this type of eating compounds the problem. Although not considered a stimulant, sugar and refined carbohydrates can interfere with sleep. A diet high in sugar and refined carbohydrates, and eating irregularly, can cause a reaction in the body that triggers the fight-or-flight response, which causes wakefulness.

Chocolate

Chocolate gives an initial sugar and caffeine buzz—a double hit! But in the end, it leaves you weary. I know when I'm stressed, I wouldn't be able to stop at one chocolate; I would look up and find the whole block or packet of chocolate biscuits have vanished. Maybe I had a chocolate-eating fairy at my house? Hmmm…It's a possibility, but I don't think so!

Salty chips dehydrate the body and brain and bring on fatigue. High-fat meals raise stress hormones and keep them high.

Sugar, nicotine and alcohol also stimulate adrenaline, another hormone released to prepare you for fight or flight. Such stimulants can trigger a stress reaction even when no major external stress is present.

A lack, as well as an excess, of blood sugar (glucose) in the body can be devastating. The body strives to maintain blood sugar levels within a narrow range through the coordinated efforts of several glands and their hormones.

After a meal, the body responds to the rise in blood glucose by secreting insulin, a hormone produced in the pancreas. The insulin lowers blood glucose by increasing the rate at which the cells throughout the body take up glucose.

Declines in blood glucose can cause the release of adrenalin and cortisol by the adrenal glands, which mirrors the effect of the fight-or-flight response. A blood sugar rollercoaster isn't only at the heart of most weight problems, it can also be a major factor in reducing our ability to cope with stress.

Managing blood glucose levels

Rainbow of foods

There are 350,000 different forms of edible plants on this planet that will assist you in managing your blood glucose levels. How many do you eat in a week? A variety is essential, as each type and colour of food contains different vitamins and minerals.

Interestingly, your body becomes stressed by trying to break down the same food over and over. So eat a 'rainbow' of food colours instead!

Drink water

To deal with stress, drink good quality filtered water. It hydrates every part of the body and brain, and helps you cope better with stressful situations. A good rule is to take a few sips every fifteen minutes. The best sources are room temperature, still water in glass or BPA-free bottles (some plastic bottles can leach chemicals into the water inside), or use a jug filter system that you fill from the tap. Do NOT use that new sexy water that's loaded with sugar. Just stick to that pure, clean filtered stuff that falls from the sky.

CTPG Oils and Aromatherapy

I've found that the CTPG metabolic blend and peppermint oil assist with my sugar cravings. When I have a few drops in a glass of water five times throughout the day, I'm not looking for all things sweet.

HOW TO REMAIN CALM IN THE MIDST OF CHAOS

"If you tell yourself you feel fine, you will."
— Jodi Picoult

Unfortunately, it's only when stress builds to depression or anxiety that people start looking for answers by referring to self-help books or going to the doctor for some medication. Anxiety and depression drugs may tone down symptoms and bring some temporary relief, but they won't address the underlying cause. The side effects can be as debilitating as the problem, such as insomnia, lack of sex drive, nausea, diarrhoea, decreased appetite and erectile dysfunction.

The common theory behind these medications is that the body has a chemical imbalance, and the drug will rebalance it. Yet neuroscience clearly shows that changing your behaviours can rebalance your brain chemicals in many cases.

Most people can overcome anxiety and depression in one to two weeks by learning and employing a number of tools and strategies that result in a lifelong, positive drug-free change.

Your sense of smell is your most primal sense and exerts surprising influence over your thoughts, emotions, moods, memories and behaviours. Scents are experienced long before anyone speaks a word.

This is why it's nearly impossible to describe them with language. Olfaction is different from your other senses, because it's processed through various pathways in your brain.

For other sensations such as sounds and visual images, sensory input is delivered straight to your thalamus, which you can think of as 'the big switchboard' in your head. From there, data goes out to your primary sensory cortices.

4 : FOOD FOR THOUGHT

However, smells are different. Before reaching your thalamus, they first wind their way through other regions of your brain, including areas controlling memory and emotion. Therefore, with scents there's all of this extra processing before you even have conscious awareness of the scent.[1]

For this reason, scents can have a powerful influence over how you think, feel and behave. Aromatherapy allows you to harness the olfactory power of plants for healing or simply enhance your state of well-being.

Essential oils carry biologically active volatile compounds in a highly concentrated form that can provide therapeutic benefits in small amounts. Please understand that I'm referring to Certified Pure Therapeutic Grade essential oils from plants, NOT synthetic fragrances and perfumes, which can be toxic and are typically loaded with allergenic compounds.

Scents can actually change your nervous system biochemistry. A Japanese study found that inhaling essential oils could modulate your sympathetic nervous system activity. Certain oils were found to be stimulating, while others were calming. For example:

Black pepper, fennel and grapefruit oil caused a 1.5-to 2.5-fold increase in sympathetic nervous system activity (as measured by an increase in systolic blood pressure).

Rose and patchouli oil resulted in a forty percent decrease in sympathetic nervous system activity.

Pepper oil induced a 1.7-fold increase in plasma adrenaline concentration, while rose oil caused adrenaline to drop by thirty percent.

Other oils have been shown to measurably decrease stress hormones, such as lavender and rosemary. Inhaling them can reduce cortisol levels.

As mentioned earlier, scents play a powerful role in memories, especially emotional ones. Olfactory input is routed through your amygdala

---

[1] http://articles.mercola.com

and hippocampus (which process emotion), but bypasses the brain's higher cortical areas, otherwise known as the 'thinking parts'.

Aromatherapy can be a beneficial adjunct to your overall health plan. It's not a replacement for wise lifestyle choices like good nutrition and exercise, but it is an excellent way to further enhance your physical and emotional health.

It's one more device you can keep in your tool bag for managing everyday stress, balancing out mood swings and improving your sleep. Your nose is an underappreciated resource, so perhaps it's time to make use of it!

Some of my favourite mood management blends are:

Grounding Blend
This blend brings a feeling of calmness, peace and relaxation. It can aid in harmonising the various physiological systems of the body and promote tranquillity and a sense of balance.

Restful Blend
This blend contains essential oils that are often used to help calm and soothe stress, overexcitement and anxiety, by helping maintain the natural state of health in the body.

Invigorating Blend
This aroma is sweet and satisfying. It's a uniquely exhilarating blend that brings together all of the uplifting and stress-reducing benefits of citrus essential oils.

Joyful Blend
This uplifting blend of oils creates an energetic aroma that can help stimulate the body's chemistry when you feel lethargic or sad.

These blends have an amazing effect on the body and are of great benefit for a wide range of issues, from learning challenges to stress

4 : FOOD FOR THOUGHT

overload. The single oils are also extremely beneficial, and it gives you the ability to create your own blends as your need arises.

You can use these oils topically or aromatically diffused in the air with an ultrasonic diffuser for the best aromatic benefit.

There's so much scientific information around that can assist and empower you in bringing balance back into your life.

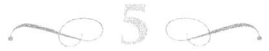

Is Your System Overdue for a Tune Up?

Most of us have experienced knowing our car isn't running well. One reason could be that the timing is off. This means the spark plugs aren't firing in a synchronised manner. The car still runs, just not at peak performance.

This is also true for our bodies. When the autonomic nervous system, hormonal system and immune system aren't working in a synchronised manner, the body doesn't work as well as it could.

We fix our car by adjusting the timing so that the spark plugs fire in the proper order and synchronisation. We can re-synchronise our body systems by creating a state of coherence and thus improving our mental focus, emotional stability and physical resilience. This allows us to operate in a more efficient manner in all areas of life.

There's a nervous system pathway that carries signals from the heart to the brain, as well as one that carries messages from the brain to the heart. Surprisingly, the heart sends more signals to the brain than the other way around!

In a way, it could be said that the heart and the brain 'talk' to one another, and together they communicate with the body. The signals they send, whether harmonious or chaotic, can make all the difference in how we feel and act.

Jagged and irregular heart rhythms send a message to the brain that indicates we're out of sync, while smooth, harmonious heart rhythms send a signal that everything is okay and working in harmony.

These messages are sent through the nervous system pathway. Nerve impulses from the heart are received at the medulla, the brain's first level, before moving up to the brain's higher centres, the amygdala, the second level, and the thalamus, the third level, which affects how we feel, think, perceive and perform.

The pattern of the signal tells the amygdala what the heart and body are experiencing, while the third brain, the thalamus, monitors the amygdala and categorises and names the feelings of joy, fear, anger or appreciation.

> *"Appreciate every little beautiful moment in every day of your life. Give it a try, and you'll see the world from another perspective."* — Thea Kristine May

When we imagine we're breathing through the area of the heart and generating a positive feeling like appreciation, we can actually change the signals the heart sends to the brain, which influences the brain's perception, thus improving how we feel.

5 : IS YOUR SYSTEM OVERDUE FOR A TUNE UP?

Another important pathway is mainly related to the activity of the third brain, the thalamus, and our ability to think clearly. When the heart's signals to the thalamus have a jagged and irregular pattern, they interfere with the ability of the thalamus to function. This results in what's called *cortical inhibition*.

In this state, the brain isn't working as well as it should; your reactions are slowed, and you can't think as clearly. This is why when you get anxious, angry or upset, you can make poor decisions and take actions you later regret.

You may ask yourself, *What was I thinking; what happened?* The answer is that the stressful feeling caused the signals in your nervous system to get out of sync, creating disordered heart rhythms and reducing your brain and body's ability to perform well.

Over time, your body gets accustomed to being discordant, and retraining is necessary to get back into sync and be coherent.

What is coherence?

Coherence is a highly efficient psycho-physiological state where all of the systems of the body work together in harmony.

Coherence is also a natural state, which can occur spontaneously, especially when we're feeling positive and upbeat or doing something we truly enjoy. However, for most people in today's high-stress world, it's rare for sustained periods of coherence to occur without practising techniques like **Quick Coherence**.

The Quick Coherence or Freeze Frame technique, developed by Doc Childre at HeartMath, is a simple and effective way to bring your body systems into synchronicity.

This technique is both simple and powerful.

You need to take deep breaths in and out, focusing on the heart area, while simultaneously concentrating on a positive emotion or a place where you feel safe. Then as you continue breathing, you'll notice the change in your physiology. *(See Diagram 3.)*

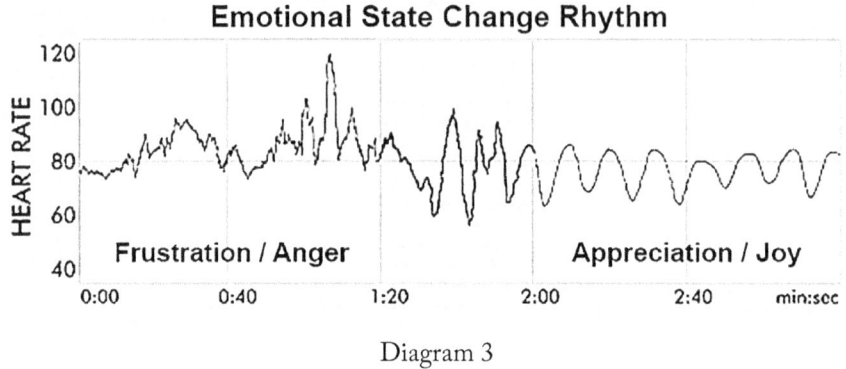

Diagram 3

"Entire waters of the Sea cannot sink a ship unless it gets inside the ship. Similarly, negativity of the world cannot put you down unless you allow it to get inside you"
— Anonymous

Quick Coherence Exercise

Acknowledge your feelings as soon as you sense you're discordant or engaged in common stressors such as frustration, impatience, anxiety, overload, anger, being judgmental or mentally gridlocked.

Take a short time out and do heart-focused breathing, which is a little deeper and slower than usual, and done through your heart or chest area.

This is proven to help create coherent wave patterns in your heart rhythm, which helps restore balance and calm in your mental and emotional nature, while activating the affirming power of your heart.

During the heart-focused breathing, imagine with each breath that you're drawing in a feeling of calm, compassion, peace, appreciation and gratitude, while making a sincere effort to activate a positive feeling.

It's scientifically proven that radiating love and self-care through your system activates beneficial hormones and boosts your immunity.

Practising will increase your awareness of when the stressful emotion has calmed into a state of ease.

The mind and emotions operate on a vibrational level. Slowing down the stressful vibration helps re-establish the cooperation and balance between heart, mind and emotions, much like an old electric fan that rattles until you turn it to a slower speed and restore the unbalanced vibration.

When the stressful feelings have calmed, affirm with a heartfelt commitment that you want to anchor and maintain this state of coherence as you re-engage in your projects, challenges or daily interactions.

Time for Reflection

Pick one day of the week as your 'Coherence Day' and practise the steps every hour or sooner, if you feel stress building.

Notice how your energy was throughout the day.

Did you have more or less stressful feelings?

What did you notice about your body?

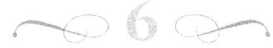

Shifting Sizes

Time and time again, I've followed the latest weight loss program. I think I would have almost tried them all, from the expensive to the not so expensive. I discovered with most of these programs and plans that they do work, and I do lose the weight, thus succeeding in my goal to shed the extra kilos.

However, what I also found was that by not dealing with the underlying issues at hand, the stress was still dominating. So back on the merry-go-round I went, again and again.

I lost the weight and back it came again, sometimes much faster than it went off. Frustrated and demoralised, I felt like I'd wasted a load of time and money. And to top it off, I missed out on some yummy foods! The clothes in my wardrobe would range from a size ten to sixteen, with a business suit to fit any body size.

I was doing stress or 'emotional' eating', making poor food choices, and even putting on weight when not overeating. I could stay on the eating program for weeks and lose weight, and then it would begin to fizzle out. Why is that?

The biggest mistake with weight-loss programs

It's ironic that the most dangerous and common mistake people make when embarking upon a health or weight-loss program has *nothing* to do with diet or exercise!

A crushing weight of both scientific and anecdotal evidence tells us that the most important determining factor in health and weight is not what you eat, or how much you exercise, or even your DNA. It's your subconscious belief systems.

Indeed, a *lack of proper emotional clearing* is the most dangerous and common mistake you can make when it comes to your health or weight.

Have you ever wondered why every time you try to embark upon a new diet or exercise program, something comes up that sabotages your progress?

Have you ever wondered why some people can eat all the wrong things and stay healthy and thin, while others gain weight just by looking at the dessert tray?

The answer is the same: subconscious belief systems.

Experts now agree that about 75 percent of overeating is emotional eating, which means that many of us are using food to cope with feelings. In today's high-stress society, many of us, both adults and children, eat high-fat or high-sugar foods to soothe emotions or relieve stress and anxiety.

In Chapter 4, we looked at what the implications of these foods were. One of the reasons why there's more emotional eating today is that people are pressed for time and under a lot of pressure. In today's fast-paced

6 : SHIFTING SIZES

world, most of us carry a lot of emotional 'loads' that add 'weight' to our lives, making it harder to stick to any diet. On top of that, being overweight or being unable to lose weight is one of the biggest causes of emotional stress in its own right.

If you're anything like me, when you're feeling a bit heavy you may look at yourself in the mirror every morning and say, 'Today I'm going to start losing fifteen kilograms'. Then by midmorning the resolve has gone, and you start feeling guilty when you eat that unhealthy midmorning snack. This causes you to feel helpless and maybe even eat more and get more stressed out and depressed. You then keep berating yourself and get into a self-loathing loop.

"To the body, obesity is not a problem, it's a solution to a problem." — Christiane Northrup

Your emotions: The key

Well, I'm excited to say that after further delving into the human psychology and how the emotional-metabolic system works, I discovered tools that can be used to address the missing factor in weight management: our emotions.

We can learn how to manage our emotional energies and release our stress without depending on food to make us feel better. The great news is that you don't have to focus on what you eat but on what you *feel*. This means no food lists or exercise regimens. Whilst these are important aspects in reducing weight and improving health, researchers have found that regulating your emotions is the first and most important aspect of weight management.

HOW TO REMAIN CALM IN THE MIDST OF CHAOS

Learning how to recognise and shift your emotions is an often-overlooked key to success in weight loss and will help other areas of your life as well, including relationships, health and quality of life.

"Between stimulus and response, there is a space. In that space is our power to choose our response. In our response lies our growth and freedom." — Victor Frankl

---

Food anesthetises your feelings in the same way as alcohol, drugs and smoking does. By someone telling you to go on a diet, they're saying to you, 'I'm going to take away the thing that makes you feel better'.

Then you come up with excuses not to lose the weight by attaching an emotion to it.

'I'm afraid to drop the weight, because then I'll feel exposed.'

'I'm afraid if I lose the weight, someone's going to notice me and say XYZ.'

'I'm afraid it will remind me of 1999 when someone attacked me.'

There are thousands of examples. Everybody has his or her own emotions to use as a reason for not losing weight.

What would make you scared to lose the weight? The initial reaction of many people is, 'Oh, don't be silly. I'm not afraid'. Well, you are, or else you would have achieved your goal and wouldn't have compelling cravings, which feel like actual cravings, like for chocolate, but they're not. They're stress-induced. Your body and chemistry are saying, *Eat the cake*, so you don't have to feel the pain, loneliness and terror that's been brewing in your body and mind for anywhere from a day to a decade.

What exactly is emotional eating? In a nutshell, it's not eating because you're hungry, but because it provides emotional and physical benefits beyond nutrition.

6 : SHIFTING SIZES

The six most common reasons you may eat emotionally are:

You're tired
When you get tired, one of the mechanisms your body uses to keep you alert and awake is to become hungry. However, eating when you're tired is dangerous, because the body's mechanisms that signal when you're full and should stop eating are impaired. The solution is to take a catnap or walk around the block, or even better, do emotional clearing on the reasons you're tired in the first place!

You're stressed
When you're stressed, your body craves carbohydrates, specifically the high-glycaemic index kind, such as sugars and processed snacks. These carbs tend to make you feel temporarily calm. In addition, chronic levels of high stress increase the production of cortisol, which locks down your body's fat stores and makes it more difficult for you to burn fat.

Emotions
It's also common to use eating to process intense emotions, which may be either negative (such as fear, anger, and jealously) or positive (such as joy and gratitude).

Emotional clearing can eliminate the underlying reasons why you feel the need to turn to food when feeling stressed or dealing with powerful emotions. In fact, high levels of stress, fear, anger and other negative emotions is one of the primary reasons people turn to emotional clearing techniques.

You're bored
Eating is a pleasurable distraction. I know from personal experience that eating while bored is a particular problem for those who suffer from serious injuries or illnesses, as often it's the only pleasure available. Because

boredom at its core is really an addiction to distraction, emotional clearing can be extremely effective at transforming the experience of boredom, so you don't need your mind constantly distracted and engaged.

Once you've done proper emotional clearing to make silence and stillness okay, boredom won't be a problem. Nor will it be necessary to eat to entertain yourself or give yourself something to do.

You're thirsty

Sometimes when you feel hungry, you're actually thirsty. The body uses hunger when it's dehydrated to get you to consume water in the form of food. Staying well hydrated will not only keep you healthier but also reduce hunger.

It's truly amazing how easy it is to confuse thirst with hunger! If you feel hungry, think about how much you've eaten recently. If it doesn't make sense that you would be hungry already, then you're almost certainly thirsty. Therefore, the next time you feel the urge to have a snack, drink some water instead, and in five or ten minutes, you may notice the hungry feeling is gone entirely.

It's a habit

We all sometimes fall into the habit of eating certain things, or at certain times.

Clear the belief systems underlying these habits, and watch your life transform!

The single most common emotional reason for carrying excess fat is an underlying subconscious fear of intimacy. By adding excess fat, you can feel like you're making yourself less attractive to potential romantic partners, thus eliminating the threat of betrayal, abandonment or in general someone hurting after you've let them get close. Victims of sexual abuse and sexual assault also commonly add a lot of excess fat for the same reason: it serves to protect them from the danger of being intimate (physically and/or emotionally) with others.

6 : SHIFTING SIZES

As long as you have powerful belief systems that tell you it's dangerous to be attractive or thin or healthy, you will sabotage your ability to do what you know you need to do to get healthy and in great shape. This sabotage may happen either consciously or unconsciously.

For example, you may knowingly sabotage your progress by choosing to eat donuts late at night, or never doing exercise, or by ordering some new diet program or supplement and never using it.

Unconscious sabotage, however, can be even more powerful and difficult to work with, as you can't overcome it with willpower alone. For example, you may commit yourself to a new exercise program, only to suffer an injury that prevents you from working out. Or you may invest in a personal trainer or a gym membership, and then suddenly lose your job or need to move out of town.

The only way to ensure you don't keep sabotaging your progress is to clear the underlying subconscious belief systems that tell you it's dangerous or uncomfortable to be healthy, lean and attractive.

There's no cookie-cutter solution here; every person's experiences will be different. But we can all use emotional clearing to eliminate the underlying, subconsciously held belief systems and traumas that make us afraid of intimacy.

Just getting people to the point where they realise their weight is serving a function, and their body is using that weight to help protect them, is a huge step.

While emotional clearing alone doesn't always cause an immediate loss of body fat, it can greatly facilitate a permanent and enjoyable lifestyle transformation to weight release and improved health by:

- healing destructive patterns of emotional eating
- releasing subconscious blocks (such as fear of intimacy) to being healthy and in great shape

- healing food allergies and sensitivities
- preparing the body for gentle and effective cleansing
- overcoming resistance to exercise
- increasing your level of commitment to your program
- healing any health problems that prevent you from taking full advantage of the cleansing, eating and exercise program

The premise of emotional clearing is simple: you contain 'subconscious software' inside of you that works through the Law of Attraction to literally attract and create every experience in your life.

This software consists of belief systems or programs you've picked up from many areas of your life that may stem from childhood experiences and DNA memories inherited from your ancestors.

The Law of Attraction works to bring you life experiences that fit your belief systems. For example, if you hold the subconscious programming, *Rich people are greedy*, you will tend to attract experiences with rich people who act greedily. Similarly, if you hold the subconscious programming, *Rich people are generous*, you will tend to attract experiences with rich people who are compassionate.

In terms of weight loss and health, if you hold the programming, *I deserve to be overweight*, it will be difficult for you to get slim. This is because you're fighting your own subconscious belief systems that makes it difficult, or perhaps impossible, to become something you don't believe you deserve to be.

Similarly, if you're a woman and have been programmed with, *If I'm thin and beautiful, I will get too much attention from men*, your subconscious will sabotage your weight loss progress, because it's trying to protect you from what it perceives to be a potentially dangerous situation.

Emotional clearing is the process of reprogramming these defective, subconscious software codes with new ones that facilitate a life of health, wealth and loving relationships. Because we all tend to attract and create our lives according to subconsciously held belief systems, you'll want to clear out the unwanted and counterproductive belief systems. Affirmations such as, *I'm afraid of being beautiful* or *Its dangerous for me to be thin* can be replaced with ones that support your goals, such as, *I deserve to be healthy and thin* and *It's safe for me to be beautiful.*

Get the Law of Attraction working for you, instead of against you, by doing emotional clearing!

What exactly is the Law of Attraction?

In short, the Law of Attraction is one of the Laws of the Universe akin to the Law of Gravity or the Law of Electromagnetism, which states that like attracts like. Yes, it really is that simple. It's based on nothing more than this basic Universal principle.

More specifically, when we talk about using the Law of Attraction to transform our lives—whether the problem is physical illness, emotional distress, poverty, dysfunctional relationships or other challenges—what we really mean is that thought energy and consciousness attracts like energy and consciousness. In other words, what we think about and put our focus on, we tend to attract to us and create in our lives.

However, unless you're one of the lucky few who can make a few tweaks to your thought patterns to heal instantly from a dreadful disease, make a million dollars or find a soul mate, you've probably found that changing your thinking and focus created, at most, small changes in your life. You made a vision board, said your affirmations and mantras, wrote out your dreams, and did all of the other popular exercises that the Law of Attraction industry recommends.

Nevertheless, it probably didn't work! If you're not a completely healthy millionaire reading this book with your loving life partner, while sipping a tropical drink at a vacation resort, clearly there's more to it than what you were told.

After taking all of the steps the book told you to do, and only seeing peripheral changes, you probably got frustrated with it after a while, since it didn't give you the results you desired.

I completely understand, as I went through all of this myself. The reason that traditional applications of the Law of Attraction such as positive thinking, affirmations, mantras, vision boards and power words are often ineffective, is simple:

They only involve the conscious mind.

In the next chapter, I'll be going into more detail about how you can harness the subconscious mind to achieve your goals.

Hint: Before eating a meal or creating an affirmation, practice the Quick Coherence Technique.

Time for Reflection

What are some goals you've been trying to achieve for a number of years and just haven't been able to break through and sustain?

What thoughts (negative/positive) and/or past events come to mind when you write your goals?

7

Harnessing the Subconcious Mind

The human mind can be divided into two sections: the conscious mind (everything that you're aware you're doing), and the subconscious mind (everything that happens without thought or any conscious effort on your part).

Your subconscious mind operates systemically, because otherwise you'd be dead. It's not random, spontaneous or flexible. Unlike your conscious mind that shifts and vacillates many times a day, your subconscious mind is fixed.

For the purpose of this book, I'm treating the subconscious mind as all of the aspects of the mind that aren't the conscious mind.

While there are some who call it the unconscious mind, and others might subdivide the subconscious into the subconscious, unconscious and super-conscious, I'm going to lump it all into the generic term, *subconscious*.

The subconscious includes the body's cellular intelligence, genetic memories and other influences of which you may not be consciously aware.

Psychologists tell us again and again that this understanding of subconsciousness is not new science. There's well-established, well-researched science over generations that verifies we establish our belief systems by the age of eight. You read that right. Not eighty. Eight. If you have a child under ten, you know how smart those kids are. What you don't think they absorbed, they absorbed big time.

This means by the age of eight, if you'll become a positive or negative person is already established. Does this thought frighten you?

Whether you'll be a confident, risk-taker or a timid, play-it-safe type is also decided at this time, as well as if you're going to be caring or selfish, open or closed-minded, your attitude toward other people, races and genders, your attitude toward money and authority, and even your attitude toward being polite and having manners and good hygiene.

Your 'programming'

Let's look at programming in computer terms. The hardware on a laptop is similar to your physical body. Inside of you, invisible and making no sound that anyone can hear except you, is your software. That programming is old, because it was placed there in the most formative stage of your life (0–8) when you had the least resistance to what anyone told you.

How often is our software updated on our operating systems? Not often. That's why you can be 28, 38 or 48, and if someone asks you:

- Do you know why you're like that?'
- Why do you always do that?'
- Why do you always overreact in that situation?
- Why do you always feel threatened?
- Why do you always have to say something cynical and have the last word?

7 : HARNESSING THE SUBCONCIOUS MIND

- Why do you always have that attitude towards that person?
- Why do you always battle with insecurity?

…with hand on heart, your answer will often be, 'I don't know why I'm like that', and you're being serious. You honestly don't remember choosing to be a certain way. You just naturally are in the flow, and it feels comfortable to you on some level, as it's familiar.

Why do any of us do or say the things we do or say? Because of subconscious programming.

How it works

When we're developing a belief system or programming the subconscious mind, we're not aware it's taking place. Everybody who's ever lived has been in conflict with what we're battling now, in the twenty-first century. People have always had two minds: conscious and subconscious.

The idea is that those two minds work together to get you where you want to go. You can have a thought in your conscious mind of something you'd like to do, but if your subconscious programming is the opposite, you're not going to go where your head wants to take you. Instead, you'll live in this constant frustration, thinking, *I know what I'd like to do, but I can't seem to do it or be there or stay there or sustain that.*

When you're a child, you don't sit down with your parents and say, 'Okay, I like that, but I don't like that. Uh, I'm going to think about that … Give me another couple of years'. You just take in the good and the bad. Whatever you see modelled, and your parents may say about the rules, your shoulds and shouldn'ts, often travel with you through to your adult life.

What's more difficult to track or trace is the information that gets through to our young, tender mind, of which there's no voice attached. It's by culture and context and environment that we're being dramatically shaped for the rest of our lives.

An iceberg provides a great analogy for the connection between the conscious and the subconscious mind, with its small visible part above the surface, and the huge part below. The conscious mind is responsible for our awareness in the waking state. Thinking analytically, creating logical order, wondering about cause and effect and asking 'why' are all characteristics of the conscious mind. It's the place of cognitive learning and understanding and uses intellect to come up with logical solutions for problems. It makes choices based on facts and moves the body deliberately.

The subconscious or unconscious mind usually operates below the level of our normal consciousness. Like in the iceberg analogy, the subconscious mind is the vaster, more substantial part of our mind.

Conscious Mind 10 - 20%

- Will Power
- Long Term Memory
- Logical Thinking
- Critical Thinking

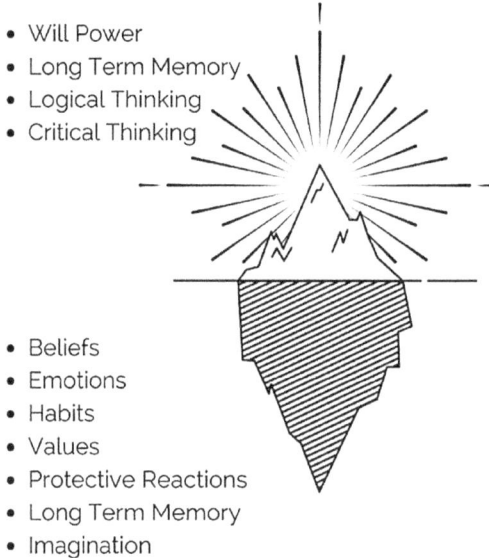

- Beliefs
- Emotions
- Habits
- Values
- Protective Reactions
- Long Term Memory
- Imagination
- Intuition

Subconscious Mind 80 - 90%

7 : HARNESSING THE SUBCONCIOUS MIND

Out of the two million bits of information that approach us every second, the conscious mind can process about forty bits of information per second; the subconscious mind can process *forty million* bits of information per second! Imagine if you could program the subconscious mind by delivering millions of instructions to it per second.

The subconscious mind is in charge of emotions, which explains why we can feel a certain way without really knowing why, or wake up grumpy one day and completely happy the next.

The subconscious mind also stores memories from any events of our past. Just take a moment and think about the house you grew up in. Before you 'visited' this place in your conscious mind, you had to access this information/memory from its subconscious storage space. However, not all memory is accessible to us; one of the so-called prime directions of the subconscious mind is to seal off traumatic events we're not ready to deal with. In addition, our deepest core beliefs, values and imprints are anchored and programmed into it.

As stated earlier, the subconscious mind is also responsible for all physiological functions of the body, such as regulating our heart rate, breathing, kidney function or digestion. The conscious mind can't make the collection of trillions of cells that comprise our body work together effectively and harmoniously.

Even 'deliberate' movement, such as walking, requires the precise coordination of many different muscles that couldn't be mastered consciously.

Along those lines, have you ever noticed that you can't really recall how you drove yourself to work or finished that sandwich while watching TV? The subconscious mind takes control of these automatic movements and patterns, without our conscious awareness. In fact, studies suggest that more than 75 percent of our daily activities are regulated by the subconscious mind.

The conscious mind is a rational mind. It operates through the five senses and rationalises all that's going on. The subconscious mind is totally irrational. It will take you towards an iceberg, if that's what you choose to do, because it merely does what you ask of it.

What's so scary is that eighty to ninety percent of our mental life is subconscious, which means if we don't master it, we will constantly wrestle to get it to in flow with the ten to twenty percent we understand. This is why when we want something in our head, we can't follow through in our heart.

Dr Friedemann Schaub of Cellular Wisdom suggests that due to the 'power and enormous potential' of the subconscious mind, we can create long-lasting changes on a mental, emotional and physical level.

Once you have your subconscious mind working for you, you'll be surprised by the ease with which you achieve goals you once believed unattainable.

The subconscious mind can't process negatives. It has no filter; it just takes everything at face value.

It interprets everything you think as a positive thought. So if you think, *I don't want to be poor*, your subconscious mind focuses on the word poor, and because it doesn't do negatives, the thought becomes, *I want to be poor*, which then becomes the goal. And like a young child desperate to please, your subconscious mind will help you behave in a way that will keep you poor, which is the opposite of what you wanted!

Several areas are programmed into the subconscious mind around money.

This is why it's so important to state your goals in the positive. In this instance, instead of thinking, *I don't want to be poor*, you'd change it to, *I am wealthy*.

According to Theta Healing practices, the subconscious mind can be divided into these four levels:

The Core Level
This includes all of your experiences and memories from your current lifetime, with events that happened in your early childhood typically being the most powerful.

The Genetic Level
This level includes all of your experiences and memories of your genetic ancestors, back through the generations.

The History Level
This level consists of the beliefs and experiences carried over from previous lives, the history of your race and collective consciousness.

The Soul Level
This level is the 'big picture' as to why you're physically here on Earth.

Your subconscious thrives on new experiences. It's like a mischievous monkey; it will get you into trouble if you don't keep it from getting bored.

You can find constructive ways of keeping your mind occupied such as reading, doing puzzles or taking up a hobby. Activities like these will make your brain cells grow more physical dendrites (the branches of a brain cell) and keep you mentally fitter. For calming your mind, keeping stress levels at bay and increasing your creativity, there's nothing better than the Quick Coherence Technique.

The subconscious mind will keep you on the straight and narrow path of whatever morality it's learned by enforcing its morality on you, even if society judges that morality wrong.

For instance, terrorists will kill and destroy without qualms, because their moral code teaches that they're a freedom fighter, so they believe they're actually being moral by fighting against a society with conflicting beliefs to their own. A gang member may kill to protect the honour of their gang without feeling any guilt, because they've learned that gang honour is more important than the commandment, *Thou shalt not kill*, or even the risk of imprisonment due to breaking the law.

If, on the other hand, your subconscious decides that you deserve to be punished, you will be wracked with guilt and exhibit behaviours designed to punish yourself, even though no laws exist that state what you did deserves punishment.

You can change these patterns.

HOW TO REMAIN CALM IN THE MIDST OF CHAOS

Essential Oils Toolkit:

For releasing: Lemongrass (The Oil of Cleansing), Renewal Blend and Cilantro (The Oil of Releasing Control).

For manifesting good outcomes: Wild Orange (The Oil of Abundance), Patchouli (The Oil of Physicality) and Ginger (The Oil of Empowerment).

"You can create with both your conscious and subconscious mind, and your mind is able to transform your life much more quickly and much more powerfully when your entire mind, conscious and subconscious alike, is aligned to achieve the same purpose." — Anonymous

---

Time for Reflection

What patterns do you see repeating in your life?

Do you have feelings of embarrassment, shame and sometimes guilt?

Ask yourself, *What am I holding onto from the past?*

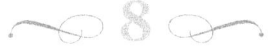

Emotions! Are They Overrated?

---

*"Positive emotions can have effects beyond making people
'feel good' or improving their subjective experiences of life.
They also have the potential to broaden people's habitual
modes of thinking and build their physical, intellectual
and social resources.
These processes can help people overcome current stresses
faster and make them more resilient to future adversities."*
— *Barbara L. Fredrickson*

HOW TO REMAIN CALM IN THE MIDST OF CHAOS

Do you have a cupboard or drawer in your home where you stash stuff in a hurry when you're preparing for the arrival of guests or cleaning the house for a much-anticipated party? Most of us have junk drawers or odds-and-ends storage areas. We store stuff until the day comes when we can't get the drawers shut or keep the door closed.

The same is true for our emotional lives. If a person keeps stuffing unaddressed emotions down year after year, the day will come when those buried emotions come pouring out.

So let's take a closer look at emotions and how they work.

Through the years, the scientific studies linking emotions to disease have produced an impressive body of research, all of which points to the conclusion that both the good in our lives and the dis-ease are the result of mental thought patterns.

For years, the Institute of HeartMath has done some of the best alternative clinical research in the world. One study definitely falls into the hard-to-believe category, and yet it's true.

They placed human DNA in a test tube, had test subjects hold it in their hands and instructed them to think painful thoughts by recalling destructive memories, because it's impossible to have one without the other. Once the subjects did this, researchers took the DNA out of the test tube and examined it. The DNA had been damaged.

With the next samples, they placed a new specimen in the test tube and had the subjects think good and happy thoughts by accessing good memories, because again, they go hand in hand. Once completed, the researchers took the DNA out of the test tube, examined it and discovered there had been a healing effect on the DNA.

So what does that mean for us? The only explanation is that the activation of certain memories seems to damage DNA, while activation of healthy memories may literally heal DNA. How exciting is that?

Just how do emotions produce a physical manifestation? Let's take a look.

8 : EMOTIONS! ARE THEY OVERRATED?

How emotions affect the physical

The basic communication link between what we think in the brain, and what we experience in the cells of the body, are neuropeptides. Dr Candace Pert, a noted stress researcher, demonstrated that a certain class of immune cells, the monocytes, have tiny molecules on their surface called neuroreceptors that are a perfect fit for neuropeptides. All monocytes have these receptor sites.

The brain produces the neuropeptides, which are chains of amino acids, and conducts them along the nervous cells throughout our body. They're like the keys that fit into molecular locks of every cell. Dr Pert has also referred to them as bits of the brain floating through the body. The brain 'talks' to the immune cells, and in turn, the immune system cells communicate back to the brain, using these messengers called neuropeptides. If your brain interprets physical perceptions as anger, fear or depression, every immune cell of your body quickly understands that interpretation.

Not only do the brain and the cells of the body communicate, but they also have a degree of memory.

As featured in Chapters 3 and 4, you'll recall that stress reactions at the cellular level are pervasive and far-reaching.

An entire system of physical responses primarily involves the hormones epinephrine and norepinephrine. They have a dramatic effect on the sympathetic nervous system during periods of intense stress.

When stressful events occur, the brain perceives it and responds by triggering the release of specific hormones from the hypothalamus, pituitary gland and adrenal gland. The stress response also triggers the adrenal glands to release epinephrine, which is also called adrenaline. The sympathetic nerves are then stimulated to release more epinephrine. Since the sympathetic nerves are located throughout the body, even in the organs and tissues, it means that when they're stimulated, your heart rate increases, your colon is stimulated (which may cause diarrhoea), you sweat and your bronchial tubes dilate, allowing more oxygen to enter.

Hormones work in a precise balance in the body. The right amount of any one hormone produces positive results, but too much or too little of a particular hormone can produce negative results.

Dr Hans Selye, an endocrinologist, was one of the first researchers to link emotional stress and disease. He reasoned that fear, anger and other stressful emotions caused the adrenal glands to become enlarged by over-stimulating the pituitary gland to produce an oversupply in hormones. That rush of adrenaline (also called epinephrine) during high stress can enable the body to perform amazing feats of strength; hence, the stories of elderly people lifting objects of amazing weights to save someone or an individual taking on an army by themselves.

Adrenaline is a stress hormone that produces a high as powerful as that of any drug. It's secreted by the adrenal glands that stimulate the heart and increases blood sugar, muscular strength and endurance. Elevated levels of adrenaline can make a person feel great. With adrenaline pumping through their body, they have a lot of energy, need less sleep and tend to feel excited about life in general. Those in high-stress professions can become addicted to that stressful feeling, which is actually their own adrenaline flow.

Adrenaline is a powerful hormone that has far-reaching physical effects. It focuses the brain, sharpens eyesight and contracts muscles in preparation for fight or flight. It also causes your blood pressure and heart rate to increase, even as blood vessels constrict. When adrenaline begins to flow through the body, digestion shuts down as blood is shunted away from the digestive tract and sent to the muscle.

If the stress is short-lived, a little burst of adrenaline does more good than harm. For instance, when facing an angry dog or a sudden confrontation with an enraged person, your body will likely react to the perceived danger and stress by pumping a burst of adrenaline and cortisol into the system. This burst is usually followed by fatigue, and most likely, exhaustion.

8 : EMOTIONS! ARE THEY OVERRATED?

Remember that the body can also perceive a fight with a family member, or someone cutting you off in traffic, in the same way. It perceives danger and responds quickly.

In normal conditions, this cycle of adrenaline/cortisol and fatigue/rest in response to short-term stress, is generally harmless to the body and can potentially save your life.

However, long-term, unaddressed stress, is unhealthy. If you're living for years in a state of unresolved anger toward a spouse or child, the flow of adrenaline can become excessive. Or if you work for years under a boss or system that makes you feel powerless or abused, you may experience nearly constant anger or a sense of danger. This long-term emotional stress causes a steady flow of adrenaline and cortisol into the bloodstream, and that flow has a damaging effect on your body.

Prolonged, elevated levels of adrenaline may increase your heart rate and blood pressure to the point that a rapid heartbeat and high blood pressure become the norm. That's not good!

Elevated levels of adrenaline over time can also cause an elevation in triglycerides, which are fats in the blood, as well as an elevation of blood sugar.

It can also cause blood to clot faster (which contributes to plaquing), the thyroid to become overly stimulated and the body to produce more cholesterol. All of these effects are potentially deadly over time.

And then, there's elevated cortisol.

As previously mentioned, when the body releases adrenaline into the system, it also releases the hormone cortisol.

Elevated levels of cortisol over time cause blood sugar and insulin levels to rise and remain that way. Triglycerides increase in the blood stream and can stay at elevated levels, while higher cholesterol levels are also capable of making the body gain and retain weight, especially in the midsection.

Too much cortisol can deplete bones of vital calcium, magnesium and potassium, leading to bone density loss. In addition, too much cortisol can cause the body to retain sodium (salt), which contributes to increases in blood pressure.

Chronically elevated levels of cortisol have been shown to:

- impair immune function, which has been linked to a wide range of diseases
- reduce glucose utilisation, a major factor in both diabetes and weight control
- increase bone loss, which has implications for osteoporosis
- reduce muscle mass and inhibit skin growth regeneration, both of which are directly related to strength, weight control, and the general aging process
- increase fat accumulation
- impair memory and learning and destroy brain cells

When left unaddressed, the constant release of adrenaline and cortisol, two of the most prominent stress hormones, can damage the body similar to acid etching away at metal. Hours after a stressful situation has calmed down, these hormone levels can remain high, continuing to wreak havoc and damaging the body.

When emotional stress continues long-term and reaches a chronic level, the result of the continual production of these hormones becomes even more destructive, creating toxicity in the body. The ongoing production and infusion of these biological chemicals damages tissues and organs, and the result is that many disease forms emerge.

With the easy access to technology nowadays, premature stress levels in younger people is more predominant. The subconscious, exposed to extreme violence in various media forms such as TV and video games, doesn't know whether it's real or imagined. This means that each time we witness these images, our body jumps into the chemical reactions of the fight, flight or freeze response.

The body reacts the same to stress, whether it's a positive or negative experience; it has no filter.

8 : EMOTIONS! ARE THEY OVERRATED?

Not all stress is equal

Some emotional states cause more damage than others. The emotions of intense joy and intense grief both apply physical stress. However, intense grief is far more damaging.

We have an inbuilt stress gauge in our bodies. The emotions that cause the most damage are rage, bitterness, depression, anger, worry, frustration, fear, grief and guilt.

We need to learn how to turn off stress as we experience it. This is where the Quick Coherence Technique can be a valuable skill to utilise.

Remember that short-term stress is fine, if it's in response to an immediate danger, but long-term stress that becomes chronic will create disease in the body.

"Give your stress wings and let it fly away."
— Terri Guillemets

A trapped emotion is literally a ball of energy that can be anywhere from about the size of a golf ball to the size of a volleyball. Wherever these lodge in the body, they will distort the normal magnetic energy field, and when you distort it long enough, you end up having physical problems.

Like having decreased circulation, interference in the flow of *chi* energy obstructs the flow of the lymph and compromises your ability to get rid of toxins. Commonly what happens is that you end up having some kind of discomfort in that tissue or a malfunction in that body area, depending on where the trapped emotion lodges.

Trapped emotions can lodge in:

- the lower back, often giving you lower back pain
- in your neck, giving you neck pain

- in your uterus, so you might have a hard time conceiving
- in the liver, probably resulting in a hard time detoxifying your body, so your immune system might start to go down

Depending on where these balls of energy lodge, you can be affected physically, emotionally or mentally.

The role of energy

Physicists have proven that everything in the universe is made of energy, even down to the tiniest sub particle. They've found this to be true not only for our external world but our internal one as well.

Within our bodies we have various systems that work together to allow us to function normally. These systems are co-dependent on each other.

Our skeletal system sets the backbone for our muscular system; our muscular system works in harmony with our nervous system; and the circulatory, respiratory, endocrine, digestive, excretory, reproductive and immune systems fall into place accordingly. If one of these systems is out of balance, it impacts the entire harmony of the body.

The other system that helps to keep the body functioning at full capacity, and is often overlooked, is the energetic system.

The energetic system is made up of a magnetic energy field, or aura, that encapsulates the body and connects to all other systems.

For more than a hundred years, scientists have been investigating the existence of an aura (energy field). Christian, Buddhist, Tibetan, Native American and Celtic traditions have documented the human aura for thousands of years. We see it in artist depictions of religious paintings. In *Future Science*, by Stanley Krippner, he lists 97 different cultures that at some point reference the human aura.

In the 1930s, Russian scientist Semyon Kirlian invented a new photographic process that involved directing a high-frequency electrical

8 : EMOTIONS! ARE THEY OVERRATED?

field at an object. He discovered that not only did the auric magnetic field show up in the stills, it also changed and mutated, depending on different emotional, mental and physical states. What an amazing discovery, to actually see how the emotions impact our body.

In the late 1900s, a group of soviet scientists from the Bio-information Institute of A.S. Popow discovered that living organisms emit energy vibrations at a frequency between 300 and 2000 nanometres. They coined this energy the *biofield*.

The Science Academy in Moscow and research in Great Britain, the Netherlands, Germany and Poland, have confirmed this biofield. Numerous other experiments further exemplify the human energy field, including verifying colours, shapes and sizes depending on the person. You can often feel this when someone comes up behind you. You'll pick up their energy field before they've even entered into your conscious awareness.

From a scientific perspective, the aura, or bio-magnetic field, gives messages about events taking place inside the body that wouldn't normally read from the outside. Many alternative medicine practitioners describe it as the 'dis-ease' or disharmony in the auric field that acts as a warning sign for physical ailments and sicknesses in the physical body. Many diseases and illnesses are energetically created before they're physically manifested. This is why it's so important to proactively address your stress and emotional triggers.

We all interact in each other's energy fields every day. How we're feeling emotionally emits into the energy field, so be mindful of who you're mixing with and how you feel after leaving their company. Do you feel uplifted or deflated? Or did you experience no change?

Time for Reflection

Can you recall times that you've entered a room, and the energy feels light and uplifting?

Has there ever been a time that you left an event or location, and you felt heavy and burdened?

Forgiveness! Seriously?

"To forgive is to set a prisoner free and discover that the prisoner was you." — Lewis B. Smedes

---

Most of us carry around anger, resentment, jealousy or some other negative emotion directed towards others. Unless dealt with, these unresolved emotions will eventually broadly affect the quality of our life and those around us.

Nearly everyone's been hurt by the actions or words of another. Perhaps your mother criticised your parenting skills, your colleague sabotaged a project or your partner had an affair. These wounds can leave you with lasting feelings of anger, bitterness or even vengeance. However, if you don't practise forgiveness, you might be the one who pays most dearly. By embracing forgiveness, you can also embrace peace, hope, gratitude and joy. Consider how forgiveness can lead you down the path of physical, emotional and spiritual wellbeing.

Generally, forgiveness is a decision to let go of resentment and thoughts of revenge. The act that hurt or offended you might always remain a part of your life, but forgiveness can lessen its grip on you and help you focus on other, positive parts of your life. Forgiveness can even lead to feelings of understanding, empathy and compassion for the one who hurt you.

Forgiveness doesn't mean you deny the other person's responsibility, and it doesn't minimise or justify the wrong. You can forgive the person without excusing the act. Forgiveness brings a kind of peace that helps you go on with your life.

It cuts the emotional and energetic tie to that particular event. It's an act of will that we choose not to be connected to that hurt anymore. It doesn't remove the event from our lives or deny it happened. It just takes the trigger and the emotional pull away that keeps us connected to that person or event. It's like cancelling a debt owed to us.

When we forgive, it enables us to release any buried anger, shame, resentment, guilt, regret, hate and any other deep emotions that can make us ill physically, emotionally, mentally and spiritually.

Repeatedly getting triggered by an event that happened in the past means you need to let go, and you'll know you're successful when you have no charge around the event.

Releasing grudges and bitterness makes way for compassion, kindness and peace.

Forgiveness can lead to:

- healthier relationships
- greater spiritual and psychological wellbeing

9 : FORGIVENESS! SERIOUSLY?

- less anxiety, stress and hostility
- lower blood pressure
- fewer symptoms of depression
- lower risk of alcohol and substance abuse

One of the reasons many people find it difficult to forgive is that they have a false understanding or a fuzzy concept of forgiveness. Let me be clear about what I mean, and don't mean, when I use this word.

According to Don Colbert, M.D. (Stress Management 101 2006), forgiveness isn't based on finding some redeeming quality that makes a person worth forgiving. We can never base genuine forgiveness upon an individual's 'good behaviour' compensating for previously hurtful behaviour. Forgiveness is something that happens on the inside of you. It comes solely from your desire to forgive for the sake of forgiving.

> *"Anger makes you smaller, while forgiveness forces you to grow beyond what you were."* — Cherie Carter-Scott

The healthiest people among us seem to be generous souls who laugh easily, forget unpleasant events quickly and are swift to forgive even the gravest offenses. Childlike behaviour keeps a person unencumbered emotionally, spiritually and in the end, physically. Only genuine forgiveness can quench the hot coals of toxic emotions and allow you to live free of the searing, scarring remnants of deep inner hurt.

We must Never Lose Sight of the Fact That Forgiveness is a Matter of the Will.

When you're hurt by someone you love and trust, you might become angry, sad or confused. If you dwell on hurtful events or situations, grudges filled with resentment, vengeance and hostility can take root. If you allow negative feelings to crowd out positive ones, you'll be swallowed up by your own bitterness or sense of injustice.

By remaining unforgiving, you could pay the price repeatedly by bringing anger and bitterness into every relationship and new experience. Your life would become so wrapped up in the wrong, that you'd be unable to enjoy the present. You'd become depressed or anxious and feel your life lacks meaning or purpose, or that you're at odds with your spiritual beliefs. You could lose valuable and enriching connectedness with others.

Forgiveness is a commitment to a process of change. To begin, you might:

- consider the value of forgiveness and its importance in your life at a given time
- reflect on the facts of the situation, how you've reacted, and how this combination has affected your life, health and well-being
- actively choose to forgive the person who's offended you—when you're ready
- move away from your role as victim and release the control and power the offending person and situation has had in your life

As you let go of grudges, you'll no longer define your life by how you've been hurt, and you might even find compassion and understanding.

Forgiveness can be challenging, especially if the person who's hurt you won't admit wrongdoing or doesn't speak of their sorrow. If you get stuck, consider the situation from their point of view. Ask yourself why someone would behave in such a way. Perhaps you would have reacted similarly if you faced the same situation.

In addition, consider broadening your view of the world. Expect occasional imperfections from the people in your life. You might want to reflect on times you've hurt others and on those who've forgiven you. It can also be helpful to write in a journal, pray or use guided meditation, or talk with someone you believe is wise and compassionate, such as a spiritual leader, mental health provider, or impartial loved one or friend.

If the hurtful event involved someone whose relationship you otherwise value, forgiveness can lead to reconciliation. This isn't always the case, however. Reconciliation might be impossible if the offender has died or is unwilling to communicate with you. In other cases, it might not be appropriate. Still, forgiveness is possible, even if reconciliation isn't.

Getting another person to change their actions, behaviour or words isn't the point of forgiveness. Think of it as being about transforming your life by bringing you peace, happiness, and emotional and spiritual healing. Forgiveness can take away the power the other person continues to wield in your life.

Perhaps the most difficult act of forgiveness is forgiving ourselves. Truly being able to move forward into emotional well-being means looking at our own lives and those areas where we feel we've failed. We need to forgive ourselves. Being unable to do this can result in shame, remorse, guilt and regret.

> *"Guilt is always hungry; don't let it consume you."*
> — Terri Guillemets

The first step is to honestly assess and acknowledge the wrongs you've done and how those wrongs have affected others. At the same time, avoid judging yourself too harshly. You are human, and you'll make mistakes. If you're truly sorry for something you've said or done, consider admitting it to those you've harmed. Speak of your sincere sorrow or regret, and specifically ask for forgiveness—without making excuses. Remember that you can't force someone to forgive you. They need to move to forgiveness in their own time. Whatever the outcome, commit to treating others with compassion, empathy and respect.

Some people find it difficult to forgive themselves for the abuse they've imposed on spouses or children, extramarital affairs they've had, getting an abortion, partaking in drug or alcohol abuse, or squandering the family's money on gambling. It isn't enough to say, 'Oh well, that was in the past. I'll forget that and move forward'.

You may very well discover that once you've worked through your own process of forgiveness, you'll look back and realise that what happened to you has been turned into a blessing in your life and isn't the grievance and scar you'd initially thought it to be.

Genuine forgiveness produces healing emotions, such as love, deep peace of mind and heart, and genuine joy. Embrace the wholeness for which you were designed.

Forgiveness is the act of unchaining yourself from thoughts and feelings that bind you to an offense, imagined or real, committed against you. It's a commitment to a process of growth and change. The first step is to recognise the value of forgiveness and the positive impact it can have in your life.

When we forgive, we release the control and power of the offending person and stop playing the victim. We no longer define our lives by how we've been hurt and instead will define ourselves by how we've grown.

> "Never forget the three powerful resources you always have available to you: love, prayer, and forgiveness."
> — H. Jackson Brown, Jr.

You may have heard of Tony Buzan. He's a leading expert on human potential, and he has some fascinating information to share with us.

9 : FORGIVENESS! SERIOUSLY?

He asks us to imagine the human brain as a large neural jungle with billions and billions of possible neural networks and connections. These neurons are like a forest, and the first person who walks into this forest won't know where to go and simply has to battle through the jungle.

The second person who walks into the forest will see a small pathway.

After another ten people have walked this trail, it's become a clear, flattened pathway, which is now used by everyone. In fact, it becomes the automatic, unquestioned choice.

Our beliefs, habits and actions function in the same way; eventually behaviour becomes automatic. We can choose to start creating a new pathway in the forest at any time, and with repeated trips, can create new beliefs, habits and actions.

Essential Oils Toolkit

Essential oils that support this process are Geranium, Calming Blend, Renewing Blend and Thyme

Time for Reflection

List everything you need to let go of.

How willing are you to let go of these things? Notice your reaction to each one and write them down.

What will you have to do to let them go?

How willing are you to do so?

10

Essential Support

"Yesterday I was clever, so I wanted to change the world.
Today I am wise, so I am changing myself."
— *Rumi.*

We're living in a world of emotional chaos. An increasing number of research shows that our emotional well-being can have an extreme impact on our physical health and wellness, and that experiencing physical pain or sickness could relate to our emotions being out of balance. Now, more than ever, many experts are under the impression that stressful emotional states impact the general health of the human body.

Numerous articles mention the probability that several ailments come from emotional troubles that link back to early life, childhood and even the womb. These emotional challenges can jeopardise body systems and impact future generations, because it creates the equivalent of a molecular memory in fundamental parts and structures of the body. Desirable and undesirable events and ideas are recorded in our brain and confined into our memories all through our existence. These memories range from minor to overwhelming and have a gigantic impact on our well-being and happiness.

As stated in previous chapters, there's a lot going on in our mind. The unconscious brain and its complicated systems are constantly manipulating your thoughts. The unconscious part of your brain has a mission to keep you safe, so it's always looking for situations that are comfortable and familiar.

The irony is that even if you feel miserable in a situation, your subconscious mind feels familiar in it and therefore thinks it's safe. This means you will need to engage your conscious mind and summon the willpower to get you over that step. I would like to go into a little more detail about that now.

Your brain, the protector

Do you ever feel that you take one step forward and two steps backwards? No matter how determined you are to change, you can't seem to get ahead. Every time you attempt to do something different like getting fit, starting a new business or going exploring online for new ways to better yourself, the reptilian brain feels the need to protect you against change, which is unknown territory, and brings you back to its comfort zone.

Often, this comfort zone is actually what you're trying to change. Your logical brain says you need to alter something, but your reptilian brain says, 'Even though I feel miserable here, I feel safe, because this is what I know, and it's safer to stay with what I know.'

10 : ESSENTIAL SUPPORT

Our natural brain hasn't changed over the past 50,000 years and has only one role: to keep us safe. If in any situation this part of the brain perceives danger, it will use its incredible powers to keep you safe and secure. This could imply that, although you may feel depressed, the brain understands this condition as a safe one and will try to keep you in it.

Our feelings turn into chemical responses in our brain. Cells react to what you express and believe. New highways of information are built with new information. Body chemicals can become acidic, and the key to health is an alkaline body.

The human brain has a variety of roles and responsibilities, and it all functions as a whole to process the information it receives. The first brain accountable for processing is the reptilian brain. As mentioned in Chapter 2, this region is completely instinctual, and its primary interest is to survive. It responds to visuals or sounds and regulates most autonomic functions such as heart rate, breathing and body temperature. It's also involved in the fight-flight–freeze response. No emotions are felt here.

As you'll recall, the second brain is the limbic system, made up primarily of the amygdala, hypothalamus and hippocampus. It's described as the brain of instinct and emotion and is connected to anxiety reactions, such as freezing or fleeing.

As mentioned earlier, the interesting point about the amygdala is that it doesn't react to visuals or sound, only scent. Consequently, the use of aromas is a great way to manage fearfulness.

The hypothalamus is in charge of regulating how you react to emotions. When you're excited, thrilled or fearful, what triggers your heart to beat faster, your blood pressure to surge and your breathing to accelerate, is your hypothalamus performing its duty.

The hippocampus transforms your short-term memory into long-term memory and also assists you in restoring saved memory. Your memories trigger how you respond to the world surrounding you, along with what your emotional reactions are going to be. Your memories become a map to your brain as to how you react.

Your brain's purpose is to keep you alive. Those who've experienced trauma of any magnitude will discover that the brain can be triggered into obsessing about survival. Anxious feelings are the brain's way to protect you from an event you've experienced in the past happening again in the future. You survived that experience, and your brain has recorded it in order to protect you from experiencing it again, so you will continue to go through a replay of a sequence of events you survived. To stop the obsessing brain in its tracks, learn how to harness your amygdala with the use of CTPG essential oils.

Using CTPG essential oils as support

The supportive benefits of essential oils are unique. They can influence healing on the four realms of reality: emotional, physical, mental and spiritual. All aromas have a possible emotional impact that can get deep into the brain.

Our sense of smell is projected to be 10,000 times more powerful than our other senses. Every time we breathe in an essential oil, the chemical compounds travel through the nose, where they're registered by the senses in the olfactory membranes in the nasal lining. The odour molecules stimulate this lining of nerve tissues and provoke electrical stimulation to the olfactory bulb in the brain, which then transports the impulses to the amygdala, where emotional memories are kept, as well as to other areas of the limbic system. The amygdala performs a significant function in keeping and eliminating emotional distress.

Essential oils allow us to reconcile collected moments and restrained emotions, so we can accept and implement or emit them.

Emotion is the experience of energy travelling through our system. Emotional power functions at a greater pace than thought. A smell can stimulate a memory in milliseconds, while thought and visuals can take seconds.

10 : ESSENTIAL SUPPORT

High frequency, pure essential oils can unlock the subconscious entries and disengage the obstacles that keep us from eliminating our traumas. The oils oxygenate the cells and bring blockages to the surface, so they can be eliminated. The oil molecules are the tiniest molecules of all matter. Some oils even have the ability to permeate the Blood Brain Barrier.

In Chapter 8, the impact of the energy of stress and emotions on our organs was discussed. A deeper reason for this is found in the fact that every organ of the human body carries a vibrational frequency. So does each emotion. The amygdala transmits the emotion to be filed to an area of our body that complements the particular vibrational frequency of that emotion. This is why we carry anger in the liver, stress in the stomach and fear blockages in the kidneys.

Those feelings not handled at some point, resurface to provide further opportunity to learn from them. The blockages stored in our organs reduce our body's vibrational frequency, and when this falls, we're more prone to illness.

Essential oils hold electrical charges, typically electrons or negative ions, which are therapeutic and beneficial. These powerful tools, added into your daily routine, help you move through what's creating chaos in your life. The chemical makeup of your essential oils , as well as the quality, are important. Not all are created equal.

The location a plant source is grown is vitally important to its chemical composition potency. The two chemistry components with doing this healing work are *sesquiterpenes* and *monoterpenes*, which are found in a range of oils.

Sesquiterpenes are significant in the elimination of cellular blockages and have remarkable anti-inflammatory attributes. The oils that are high in sesquiterpenes are:

- Black Pepper
- Myrrh
- Ylang Ylang

- Cedarwood
- Patchouli
- Ginger
- Sandalwood

Oils that contain sesquiterpenes are soothing, both physically and emotionally.

Monoterpenes are the most compact molecules in aromatherapy that travel quickly to the nose and are fast to evaporate. Citrus oils, in most cases, have high monoterpenes and are well known for their uplifting benefits. Examples of citrus oils are:

- grapefruit
- lime
- lemon
- orange
- bergamot

Douglas Fir and White Fir are also high in monoterpenes.

Science shows us that using essential oils topically and aromatically can make a big impact on brain function and stress management, naturally enhancing physical and cognitive performance, and thus improving our quality of life and longevity.

11

What is Lurking in our DNA?

Have you been struggling for ages to achieve your personal or business success, even though you've been doing personal development for years and tried lots of processes, tools and programs? Well, it's time to discover the real reason: inherited generational emotional issues!

Have you been told that you have your dad's temper or your mum's pride or your grandma's anxiety? Well, now there's a new way to explore being free of those inherited traits and characteristics: Emotional Clearing.

Getting rid of your trapped emotions can help you overcome the obstacles of your past and bring new life to your marriage, family, and other personal relationships.

Inherited Trapped Emotions

As I discussed in Chapter 8, an Inherited Trapped Emotion is like any other trapped emotion, except it originated not from you but from an ancestor. The term inherited means it was passed on genetically.

The process is similar to inheriting DNA and other genetic material. For example, you can only inherit your hair or eye colour from a biological parent. Inherited emotions are the same. You see, things like emotions can get stuck in the family tree, so we can inherit fears, characteristics, traits, phobias, hurts and sorrows.

We can also inherit great things, too, like our grandfather's sense of humour, which we usually want to keep. But it's the negative ones we don't want to pass on, that we wish to release. Through twenty-first century means, such as amazing energy-healing technologies and the power of utilising intention, we can clear those trapped energies for good.

When do we inherit emotions?

They're inherited at the moment of conception. When the sperm and egg unite, and fertilisation occurs, a trapped emotion is passed from the parent to the fertilised egg and becomes part of the foetus. So for example, at conception, a trapped emotion can be passed from the mother or father to that fertilised egg.

You can inherit multiple emotions from both parents, and each one is a on a different frequency. Remember, every emotion has its own specific, unique frequency.

The genealogy of inherited, trapped emotions is that they can be passed down many generations, much like a family gene tree. However, like recessive genes, not all descendants will inherit the emotion. For example, you may have inherited an emotion of stubbornness from your great-grandfather, and yet all, some, or none of your children will. You just don't know.

11 : WHAT IS LURKING IN OUR DNA?

Releasing Inherited Trapped Emotions

It's possible to release generational trapped emotions, just as you can your own personal trapped emotions, through Emotional Clearing. When an inherited generational emotion is released, it pulls that flawed thread out of the entire family tree.

How do you know if you have a generational emotional issue locked in your DNA? Well, usually there's some kind of feeling of frustration, because you've worked on an issue for a long, long time, and it still comes back to haunt you.

For instance, you might be making comments like, 'But I've changed my belief system, and I don't know why I still react the same way'. This is basically a sign saying, *Help me! I have some ancestral emotional DNA to clear.*

So if someone comes to me unable to alter their reactions and behaviour, even after changing their belief system, I know there's ancestral emotional baggage to clear. I see it in relation to money issues all the time, as well as with abuse, addictions and depression.

Most of the time these inherited emotions go back as far as 80 or 120 generations, but the biggest volume tends to be in the latest five generations.

Now, it's worth reminding you that when someone has a generational-trapped emotion, it doesn't mean everyone in that lineage carries that emotional baggage. It's the same as your kids not all having the same coloured hair. Different people inherit different cellular memories or trapped emotional DNA.

When I clear something that was created fifteen generations ago on my father's side, this emotional flaw thread is pulled out between me and the original ancestor from fifteen generations ago. At the same time, it also clears up anyone sideways on my family tree who also inherited it, like brothers, sisters and cousins. The cool thing is that the flawed thread is no longer there; it kind of transmutes or dissipates for good. This also applies to your children or grandchildren, if they inherited it as well.

That flawed thread of emotion is pulled out from anyone in your lineage who inherited it.

The other cool thing about this work is that I've met clients where their mother or sister doesn't think energy work is a good thing. They're afraid of it and think it's stepping into the dark side. But when their sister or daughter comes along and does a bunch of family healing work, the other family members, usually unbeknownst to them, wind up brighter and lighter as well. They don't know why, and don't need to on a conscious level. Their spirit, or energy, knows, because a big chunk of emotional baggage was cleared from a relative of theirs.

In my work I also see this come up in a lot of female issues, like infertility; families of women who all really struggle with female cycles, fibroids or anything to do with the female reproductive system. This area is where I've personally seen the greatest improvement so far in my health.

In my preface, I mentioned my debilitating monthly hormonal issues that were keeping me from enjoying life to the full, and were depleting my iron levels and energy every month. What we found in my ancestry was a young lady born into a family of six brothers. She resented the fact that she was a girl and couldn't enjoy the fun activities her brothers were engaged in, as each month she was afflicted with a period. Therefore, with every period, the resentment built, and her emotions around each time of the month were of disgust and disconnection to her femininity.

Since I've had my own Emotional Clearing take place, those troubles are a thing of the past; no more do I have to battle with my hormones. No pills, no surgery, just clearing the emotional energy fields around it, clean and simple.

If you go back through your family tree, with Emotional Clearing you might see many women in the lineage who had trouble with fertility and other gynaecological problems.

11 : WHAT IS LURKING IN OUR DNA?

Once you start clearing these generational women's issues, you might find emotions related to abuse, oppression and sorrow.

Once all of these emotions have been released, the women in the family will start doing better. So whether or not anyone is aware that a member of the family has been doing energy work doesn't matter, as it clears from the family line anyway. Those who happened to inherit that emotional DNA baggage will have it cleared for good.

Essential Oils Toolkit

The supportive oils for working generationally are White Fir, Douglas Fir, DNA Repairing Blend, Birch and Jasmine.

12

Tapping Into New Life

Many years ago, a good friend of mine introduced me to the Emotional Freedom Technique (EFT), also known as Tapping. It was great for many applications. Over time, I put it to the side and almost forgot about it, until I started questioning why my life wasn't as it should be. So I dusted off the technique and started to practise again, taking the time to go through and sort out my emotional binds…to great success.

Many people worldwide are experiencing poor health and a mundane and unsatisfying life. They're stuck, feeling empty, having mood imbalances, chronic aches and pains, and don't know how to change and turn it around, so they can have a more joy-filled life.

They often feel the only option available is medication to suppress their anxious feelings, dull the pain and get to sleep at night. Along with these remedies comes a string of cascading side effects that are often no better than the disease they're trying to cure, and they're caught in a cycle of discontent, depression and always feeling unwell.

If this resonates with you, I can tell you there's a simple way to help shift the trapped emotions that will assist you in turning your life around and empower you. You'll be able to reclaim your health and happiness, so you can be at your best, living a life filled with peace, joy and fulfilment every day and every moment.

With Tapping, you have in your own hands a tool that's simple for anyone to use, and best of all, it is free.

Tapping provides relief from chronic pain, emotional problems, disorders, addictions, phobias, post-traumatic stress disorder and physical diseases. It's simple and painless and can be learned by anyone. You can apply it to yourself whenever you want, wherever you are.

The healing concepts that Tapping is based on have been in practice in Eastern medicine for over 5,000 years. Like acupuncture and acupressure, Tapping utilises the body's energy meridian points. You stimulate them by tapping on them with your fingertips, which means you're literally tapping into your body's own energy and healing power.

Your body is filled with life and energy, and it's designed with the ability for self-healing more powerful than you can imagine.

So how does it all work?

All negative emotions cause a disruption of the body's energy, and physical pain and disease are intricately connected to negative emotions. Health problems create feedback to the body, physical symptoms cause emotional distress and unresolved emotional problems manifest themselves through physical symptoms.

The body's health is best approached as a whole. You can't treat the symptoms without addressing the cause, and vice-versa. Adding a Band-Aid to an untreated wound doesn't produce an environment for healing, but rather an environment of festering and bacteria. And it's the same if we don't delve deeper into the underlying emotions beneath the symptoms.

12 : TAPPING INTO NEW LIFE

Everything in the universe is composed of energy, and the body is no different. By restoring balance to the body's energy, you will mend the negative emotions and physical symptoms that stem from this energy disruption. Tapping restores the body's energy balance, and negative emotions are conquered and released.

The basic technique requires you to focus on the negative emotion at hand, which is anything that's bothering you like a fear or anxiety, a bad memory or an unresolved issue. While maintaining your mental focus on this issue, use your fingertips to tap five to seven times each on twelve of the body's meridian points. (*See Diagram 4.*)

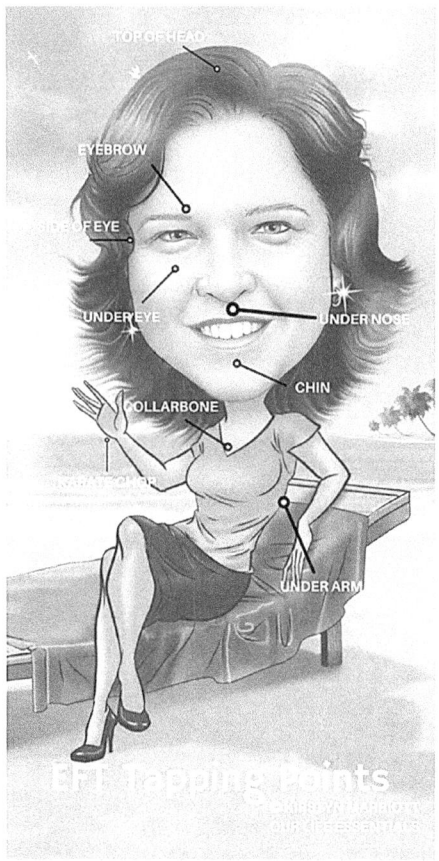

Diagram 4

Tapping on these meridian points, while concentrating on accepting and resolving the negative emotion, will access your body's energy, restoring it to a balanced state. Meridians are energy circuits throughout your body along a specific network of channels. You can tap into this energy at any point along the system.

This process is inexpensive and not time consuming, and it can be used with specific emotional intent towards your own unique life challenges and experiences.

If anything you've read in this book stirs up emotions, this technique is perfect to take the charge out of it. There are many YouTube videos on EFT/tapping and loads of resources to help you on your journey of release. Tapping and CTPG essential oils are a powerful combination in helping you release any unwanted emotional patterns.

Conclusion

In conclusion, I would like to share two truths:

1. **To heal your problems, you have to heal the relationship to stress.**
   There's just no other way. It's the one issue agreed upon in traditional health, government and alternative health research going back many years, as well as on millions of websites. You have to heal the stress if you want permanent, long-term and complete healing of your problems.

2. **To heal stress, you have to heal your memories.**
   According to numerous bodies of research, what causes the stress response in the body isn't just our current circumstances. It's our wrong or false beliefs. Those destructive cellular memories that are encoded and stored in our hearts and minds.

Is what you're currently doing working?

An experience creates an emotional reaction, either positive or negative, which then can turn into a mood. If we stay with that mood for a few hours or days, that behaviour then turns into temperament over weeks and months, until finally it develops into a personality trait. This means we're memorising our emotional reactions and living in the past, and we're basing our future on this past construct.

HOW TO REMAIN CALM IN THE MIDST OF CHAOS

We can have power over the fight-or-flight response. It can be turned on or off by thought alone, so what we're thinking regarding a future event can be a negative or positive experience. We have the power to choose. The event itself is neutral. You have the ability to transform your mind, training it to focus on the good. This can take some time if you've trained yourself to look at only the negative in life.

If you could re-live your life all over again and experience the same events, how would they look through a different set of eyes? Can you go back and see the good in life? These situations are your memories, and you can change them. You can go back in your mind and plant the outcome you desired, and then keep replaying it over and over, until you believe it happened that way, and you get the result you would have preferred.

It all comes down to whether or not you react to a situation or respond to it. Reacting means the situation has the power, while responding keeps the power within you to decide how you feel about it and how you'll deal with it.

When you see people who experience the same events, you'll notice some are devastated and never recover, while others bounce back as if it never happened. We marvel at how resilient they are, but they're just like you or me. The only difference is that they don't let the situation define them. It's just something that happened.

One of the biggest lies we've come to believe about ourselves and our true nature, is that we're nothing more than physical beings, defined by material reality, devoid of dimension and vital energy, and separate from God. To remove ourselves from the truth about our real identity not only enslaves us but asserts that we're finite beings living a linear life that lacks substance and meaning.

We're all multi-dimensional beings, with a body, mind and spirit, and if we're unbalanced in one these areas, it's like walking with two left legs; we wind up going round in circles.

CONCLUSION

Since we're wired to make habits, why not move away from the old and step into the new, with love, generosity, joy, compassion, genius and awareness?

Abandon false beliefs and perceptions, and remove layers of personal emotions you've chosen to memorise as your identity. Shed your selfish limitations.

Only you, and you alone, have the power to remain calm in the midst of chaos by choosing deliberate thought and determination. The power is yours.

Decide today, and you will transform your life.

Time for Reflection

Is it time to write that letter to someone who has hurt you, or maybe even one to yourself? Allow yourself some reflection time, and play some peaceful, relaxing music. Think back over everything you're angry about regarding yourself and others.

You may have never forgiven yourself for wetting the bed as a child and feeling the embarrassment and humiliation. That's such a long time to carry this burden! Sometimes it's so much easier to forgive others than ourselves.

Write in your letter everything you feel, and how it's affected your life.

Once you believe you've addressed all of the issues with yourself or someone else, fold the paper over and write on the outside, *It is done, it is finished, and it is forgiven. I now forgive you and set you free.*

Then burn it.

APPENDIX

To truly transform your life, you must first transform your mind.

For further information on the certified pure therapeutic grade essential oils mentioned in the book, go to:

http://www.mydoterra.com/ourlifeessentials

ACKNOWLEDGEMENTS

To my wonderful husband who has shared my stresses, and endured plenty of his own, yet still has the ability to love and support me regardless. This journey is always unfolding, and I look forward to continue sharing it with you.

To my three gorgeous children. You drive me forward to find solutions, so you can have a life of deeper understanding and success.

To my father and mother, for their unrelenting belief in me and always encouraging me to follow my path. Thank you, and I love you both. See you when it's my turn, Dad.

To Dr Caroline Leaf, for opening my mind to the wonders of neuroscience, how our internal programming can be changed and how we can choose to live life to the fullest as God intended.

To the team at HeartMath: Your ongoing research and developments have given me, and thousands of others, the tools to reduce our everyday stress impact and strengthen our resilience muscle for a longer and healthier life.

To Carolyn Cooper from Simply Healed. Without a better understanding of emotional baggage and the ability to release it at the source, life would be very different today.

To the amazing seven heart-centred owners of the largest therapeutic grade essential oil company in the world, dōTERRA: You have brought so much healing to the world with your passion for people, purity, safety

ACKNOWLEDGEMENTS

and efficiency in product, and the love and compassion you show for the amazing people who grow and harvest the precious oils. You truly are wise stewards in all senses of the term. I'm truly blessed to have had you come into my life, so I can empower others to take ownership of their health and find solutions that can change their life on so many levels. For that, I'm truly grateful.

To Bob Proctor, Dr Mario Martinez and Dr Joe Dispenza, your work has helped me break through some paradigms I didn't even know existed. Many were ingrained from cultural upbringing and created the chains that held me back. Thank you for being the change.

About the Author

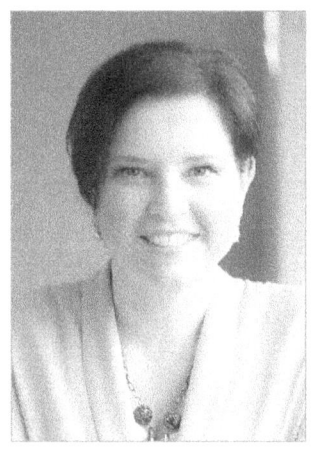

Kirstyn Marriott is a highly intelligent and motivated entrepreneur with a three-decade long business background that spans into a diverse range of fields and arenas, including banking, agriculture, property investment and events. Fulfilling predominantly leadership and training roles in working with people in organisations, Kirstyn has acquired a long list of qualifications ranging from Business Management to Project Management.

Personal stress skyrocketed during her time in the corporate world, and once the stress turned into serious physical illness, Kirstyn re-evaluated her approach to life.

Driven by her realisation of the impact our beliefs have on us, Kirstyn devoted herself to acquiring certifications in several personal development and healing methodologies before making the shift to becoming an Emotional Wellness Coach.

Kirstyn is a master of freeing people from mental, emotional and physical stress. She works with clients who are experiencing chaos and seek clarity and direction. By integrating powerful transformation methods, she's able to assist them in manifesting meaningful changes, both personally and professionally. Because of her focus on transformation on

ABOUT THE AUTHOR

all levels and in all areas, Kirstyn has been able to have a powerful impact on many lives.

Kirstyn lives in Brisbane, Queensland, Australia, along with her husband and three children. Her no-nonsense approach to helping people with self-growth enables them to quickly regain emotional clarity and direction for life.

Contact:

kirstyn@kirstynmarriott.com

REFERENCES

My sources for the quotes in this book have been many and varied, including books and online sources over many years of personal research

Murray M T 2012, **Stress, Anxiety and Insomnia** *- What the Drug Companies Won't Tell You and Your Doctor Doesn't Know, 2nd edn, Mind Publishing, Canada.*

McGee R S 2003, **The Search for Significance**, *2nd edn, Thomas Nelson Inc, Nashville.*

Don Colbert, MD, **Deadly Emotions**, *Ed. 2006, Thomas Nelson, Inc., Nashville, Tennessee*

Karol K. Truman, **Feelings Buried Alive Never Die**, *Ed. 2005*

Olympus Distributing Corporation, St George, Utah

Louise L. Hay, **You Can Heal Your Life**, *Ed. 2004, Hay House Inc, Carlsbad, California, USA*

Sara Gottfried, MD, **The Hormone Cure**, *Ed. 2013, Scribner, New York, USA*

Doc Childre and Deborah Rozman, PhD, **Transforming Stress**, *Ed. 2005, New Harbinger Publications, Oakland, California*

Doc Childre and Deborah Rozman, PhD, **Transforming Anxiety**, *Ed. 2006 New Harbinger Publications, Oakland, California*

Joyce Meyer, **Change Your Words, Change Your Life**, *Ed. 2013, FaithWords, Brentwood TN, USA*

REFERENCES

Dr Caroline Leaf, **The Gift In You**, *Ed. 2009, Improv, Northampton, MA, USA*

Jon Gabriel, **The Gabriel Method**, *Ed. 2008, Atria Books/Beyond Words, Hillsboro, Oregon, USA*

Alexander Lloyd PHD and Ben Johnson MD, **The Healing Code**, *Ed. 2013 Grand Central Publishing, New York, USA,*

Dr. Joe Dispenza, **Breaking the Habit of Being Yourself**, *Ed. 2013, Hay House, Inc, Carlsbad, California, USA*

Dr. Bradley Nelson, **The Emotion Code**, *Ed. 2007, Wellness Unmasked Publishing, Mesquite, NV, USA*

Bob Proctor, **You Were Born Rich**, *Ed. 2015, Proctor Gallagher Inst, Scottsdale, AZ*

Inna Segal, **The Secret Language of Your Body**, *Ed. 2010, Atria Books/ Beyond Words, Hillsboro, Oregon, USA*

Dale Carnegie, **How to Stop Worrying and Start Living**, *Ed. 2004, Gallery Books, Dehradun, India*

Mona Lisa Schultz MD, **Awakening Intuition**, *Ed. 1999, Potter/ Tenspeed/Harmony, CA, USA*

Dr Libby Weaver, **Rushing Woman's Syndrome**, *Ed. 2017, Hay House UK, London, UK*

Bill Harris, **Thresholds of the Mind**, *Ed. 2002, Centerpointe Press, Lincoln, Nebraska*

Emmet Fox, **Power Through Constructive Thinking**, *Ed. 2009, HarperCollins Publishers, New York, USA*

Brian Tracy, **Eat That Frog, Ed. 2006,** *Berrett-Koehler Publishers, Inc. Oakland, CA, USA*

Joel Osteen, **I Declare 31 Promises to Speak Over Your Life, Ed. 2013,** *FaithWords, Brentwood TN, USA*

Dawson Church, **EFT for Weight Loss**, *Ed. 2013, Energy Psychology Press, Fulton, CA, USA*

Amanda Porter and Daniel McDonald, **Emotions & Essential Oils**, *Ed. Fall 2015, Enlightened Alternative Healing LLC, Salt Lake City, UTAH*

www.ingramcontent.com/pod-product-compliance
Lightning Source LLC
Chambersburg PA
CBHW060456300426
44113CB00016B/2615